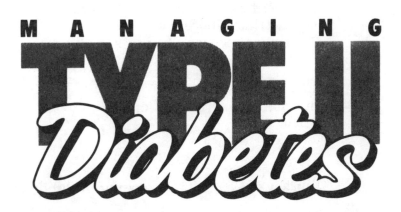

MANAGING TYPE II Diabetes

YOUR INVITATION TO A HEALTHIER LIFESTYLE

Arlene Monk, R.D., C.D.E., Sue Adolphson, R.N., C.D.E.,
Priscilla Hollander, M.D., Richard M. Bergenstal, M.D.

Cover & text design: West 44th Street Graphics
Typesetting: Shoreline Type
Printing: Precision Graphics

International Diabetes Center
©1988

Library of Congress Cataloging-in-Publication Data

Managing Type II Diabetes.

(The Wellness and nutrition library)
Includes bibliographies and index.
1. Non-insulin-dependent diabetes—Popular works.
2. Non-insulin-dependent diabetes—Treatment.
I. Monk, Arlene, et al. II. Title: Managing type 2 diabetes.
III. Title: Managing type two diabetes. IV. Series. [DNLM:
1. Diabetes Mellitus, Non-Insulin-Dependent—therapy—
popular works. WK 850 M266]
RC660.4.M36   1987   616.4′62   87-20218
ISBN 0-937721-24-7

Published by DCI Publishing
A division of Diabetes Center, Inc.
P. O. Box 739
Wayzata, Minnesota 55391

Printed in the United States of America.

ACKNOWLEDGEMENTS

We most sincerely acknowledge the help of everyone who has made this book a reality. We particularly appreciate the insights our patients have given us over the years. In addition, special thanks to:

- Those who teach and have taught in the International Diabetes Center's class, "Managing Type II Diabetes".

- Those who reviewed this manuscript: Marion J. Franz, R.D., M.S., C.D.E., and Judy Ostrom Joynes, R.N., M.A., C.D.E.

- Donnell D. Etzwiler, M.D., for his visionary leadership and commitment to education for people with diabetes and health professionals who work with those people, and his belief that people with diabetes can live well.

- The International Diabetes Center staff for their support.

- Editorial staff, particularly Donna Hoel, Lisa Bartels-Rabb, Neysa Jensen, and Michael Moore.

- The typesetters at Shoreline Type, who worked so hard to help us make our deadlines.

- The design team at West 44th Street Graphics.

- Tom Foty for his illustrations.

- The staff of DCI Publishing.

Thank you all. Without your encouragement, the task would have been much more difficult.

—The Authors

TABLE OF CONTENTS

INTRODUCTION

WELCOME ABOARD!

Almost a hundred years ago, Sir William Osler, a famous American physician, said: "The way to live a long healthy life is to have a chronic disease and take care of it."

That's certainly true for Type II diabetes. The things you need to do to take care of yourself are exactly the things all of us should always do.

Of course, no one wants a health problem—any health problem. But if you do have diabetes, we have some very good news for you.

You can be as healthy as you've ever been—maybe healthier—if you take charge and manage your diabetes to the best of your ability. We hope this book will give you the tools you need to do an excellent job.

WHAT IS IT?

Type II diabetes is a unique disorder. We don't completely understand why, but for some reason the body can't use insulin the way it should. The insulin is there—it just can't do its job. When this happens, blood glucose levels go up.

You might have heard that insulin is like a key. It attaches to body cells and "unlocks" a pathway for glucose into the cells. We could say it's like the ignition key for a car. Glucose is like gasoline. Our marvelous bodies make glucose out of food and then turn the glucose into energy. (Of course it's a whole lot more complicated. You need many other things for this all to work, but you get the point.)

If the body can't get the glucose to the places it's needed, things begin to shimmy—ever so subtly. With Type II diabetes, some glucose gets to the cells, but often not enough.

So what do we do to fix things? Since your body is making insulin, you may not need to inject more, as is the case for people with Type I diabetes. (In those folks, the pancreas can't make the insulin they need.) The job with Type II diabetes is to figure out how to help the body use the insulin already there.

At the risk of spilling the beans early, we'll give you some clues as to what we know about taking care of Type II diabetes. The greatest improvement often comes with eating the right foods and losing some weight. Exercise is the next most helpful step. Diabetes pills are the third option; they help many people. Finally, some people will need to inject insulin, but even this isn't such an awful thing to do.

We saw those lights go on when we said you may have to inject insulin. You're saying, "Now that doesn't make any sense. If you can't use the insulin already there, why inject more?" Good question. We're not sure we have a really good answer, but in some people, insulin injections do allow enough insulin to work so the blood glucose level is closer to normal.

Interestingly, meal planning and exercise seem to work very well for many people.

HOW DO YOU KNOW YOU HAVE DIABETES?

This question can have some very interesting answers. One gentleman recently told us he went to the doctor for an "ear re-check". The nurse gave him a little cup and sent him to the bathroom for a urine specimen. He did think it strange to check urine when looking in his ear seemed so onderful. (Turns logical. But modern science is strangely wout the nurse thought he said "urine check.") Anyway, the urine showed high glucose levels, which led to detection of diabetes.

Lest you feel sorry for this man, he learned a lot about diabetes, made some important changes, and probably added 10 years to his life—to say nothing of adding life to his life. He sees himself as a very lucky person.

A more typical way of discovering diabetes is through a

routine blood test. Quite often, diabetes is found when some other problem comes up—a bout of flu or an infection. Because diabetes tends to develop over a long period of time, the symptoms are often missed or are so subtle they're dismissed as a "part of growing old."

A diagnosis of diabetes is confirmed on the basis of a blood glucose test done in a laboratory. The following are the criteria identified by the American Diabetes Association for diagnosing diabetes in nonpregnant adults.

■ A random blood glucose of 200 mg/dl or higher plus classic symptoms.

■ A fasting blood glucose of 140 mg/dl or higher on at least two occasions.

WHAT ARE THE SYMPTOMS?

The classical symptoms are increased thirst, frequent urination, and unintended rapid weight loss. Vague symptoms are fatigue, frequent infections, irritability, vision changes, pain in the feet or legs, and dizziness. Most of us have one or more of these fairly often, so we tend to ignore them.

Many people have no specific symptoms at all. High blood glucose levels often are found at routine health checks in some other way—such as an ear re-check.

Now you're going to ask, if there are no symptoms, why worry about it? Well, lots of things have no symptoms and still cause problems. Not to seem trivial, but how about carpenter ants? They can sneak up on you. They get into our houses, where they gnaw at beams and studs and seldom make a sound. Once you know they're there, though, you certainly want to do something about them. So think of diabetes as carpenter ants—with a potential for eating away.

Diabetes does cause damage that often can be prevented. We've all heard horror stories about people who have lost a leg or have gone blind. This occurs because too much glucose floating around in the blood eventually damages blood vessels, starting with the most fragile ones in the eyes and feet. If you can keep glucose levels within a normal range, you stand a very good chance of avoiding those kinds of problems.

We're all different and of course there are no guarantees. But the odds are with you if you take good care of yourself.

WHO GETS DIABETES?

Actually lots of people! About 11 million in the U.S.—or about 1 in 20 people. One million have Type I diabetes—the kind that requires insulin injections for life. The other 9 million have Type II diabetes. About half the people who have Type II diabetes don't know it. Nearly half a million new cases are found each year.

Some factors do seem to lead to higher risks for diabetes. Family history is one. So don't be shy about telling your children and grandchildren and someday your great grandchildren what you learn about diabetes. You might even be tempted to encourage them to live the way you do.

Another risk factor, of course, is obesity. Our sedentary lifestyle gets us in trouble. We were never meant to sit most of the time, and our bodies pay the price.

IS IT SERIOUS?

People with Type II diabetes often think they have the mild form of diabetes—particularly if insulin injections aren't needed or if the disease is discovered well into the adult years. However, because of the risks of complications, diabetes must be considered a serious disease. The terms "borderline" or "a touch of diabetes" should not be used in place of Type II diabetes, since they imply it is not a serious condition.

WILL IT GO AWAY?

Sorry to say, no. There's no such thing as a "touch of diabetes." Nor is there "borderline diabetes." We could say it's kind of like the old "touch of pregnant" joke—but we won't. Once you've got it, you've got it.

The good news is you have lots of options for living very well with diabetes. Blood glucose levels do go up and down, and what we want is to keep those levels as close as we can to normal. It's a bit like keeping a close eye on your carburator.

Our mission in creating this book is to show you what you can do to control your blood glucose levels. We believe good control helps avoid complications associated with diabetes and offers the best chance for a vigorous, healthy life. We're going to give you lots of information about controlling blood glucose, and we hope you find it interesting and valuable as you chart your own course.

SO WHERE DO WE START?

When the Minnesota Twins won the World Series in 1987, a reporter asked a player how they did it. The player's reply: "We put on a new attitude. We believed."

That's the key to a whole lot of successes in life. A positive, hopeful, optimistic approach to managing your health is very important. Information also is vital, and that's what this book is about. We'll take you step-by-step through what you need to know and what you need to do. We believe it works.

CHAPTER 1

MORE ABOUT DIABETES

Diabetes is an ancient disease. The first description goes back about 1500 years before Christ. The name "diabetes" is from the Greek and literally means "to run through a siphon." Water seems to run right through people who have the disease.

The word "mellitus", which means "honey", was added many hundreds of years later when the early scientists recognized the high glucose levels in the urine of people with diabetes. Early historians reported that heredity was important in what they called "sweet-water disease."

About the sixth century A.D., Type II diabetes was first recorded. It originally was called "maturity onset" diabetes, since it usually occurred after age 40. In the nineteenth century, a man named Langerhans described groups of cells in the pancreas resembling little islands. He didn't know what the cells did, but his discoveries were critically important in events that followed. A few years later, two German scientists discovered when the pancreas was removed from animals, diabetes developed.

In 1921, two Canadian physicians put the puzzle together when they obtained purified, minced islet cell tissue from animals and injected it into animals with diabetes. When the blood glucose levels fell, they realized they were on to something.

Banting and Best, the Canadian physicians, are credited with saving the lives of millions of people with diabetes. Their discovery of insulin resulted in a whole new era in treating diabetes.

THE PANCREAS

The pancreas is a gland, weighing about half a pound, located just below and behind the stomach. The islets of Langerhans within the gland contain beta cells, which secrete insulin. The islets make up only about one percent of the pancreas.

Beta cells are amazing. A normal pancreas has about 100,000 islets of Langerhans, and each islet has from 80 to 100 beta cells. These cells can measure the blood glucose every 10 seconds to within a range of 2 milligrams percent. (That's mighty good!) Within a minute to a minute and a half, the beta cells can deliver the exact amount of insulin needed to keep blood glucose levels normal.

When diabetes isn't present, it's almost impossible to raise the blood glucose level too high. The insulin supply is almost inexhaustible.

The pancreas has several other functions, including producing certain enzymes needed for digestion. In addition, the pancreas contains alpha cells, which make a substance called glucagon. Glucagon seems to balance out the effects of insulin and helps keep blood glucose levels normal. Delta cells also are found in the pancreas. These cells make yet another substance, called somatostatin, which appears to carry messages between insulin and glucagon.

WHAT DOES INSULIN DO?

As we said earlier, insulin is like the key that controls storage and movement of fuel.

The body uses two types of fuel—glucose and fats. Carbohydrate is the most readily available source of glucose and can easily be converted into fuel for immediate use. Some glucose will be stored in the liver and muscles as glycogen to be used later and during exercise. Carbohydrates not needed for immediate energy or replacement for glycogen will be changed to fat. Insulin is required for each of these processes to take place.

Protein, which is made up of amino acids, can be a secondary source of glucose. If the body doesn't receive enough carbohydrate to use as a fuel source, the liver, with insulin present, can change some of the amino acids into glucose. Insulin also allows amino acids to be used for building and repairing muscle and body tissues (in other words for healing our injuries).

Fat fuel in the form of triglycerides is absorbed from the intestine. Insulin allows triglycerides to go directly into fat cells where it is stored and used for future energy needs.

Insulin, therefore, is important not only for the body's use of carbohydrates, but in the use of protein and fat as well.

WHAT HAPPENS IN DIABETES?

When enough insulin is not available or when the insulin isn't working quite right, as in Type II diabetes, the body reacts much like a machine running out of fuel. Because the fuel glucose can't get into the cells where it is needed, it builds up in the blood. The unused glucose circulates through the kidneys. When the amounts of glucose get to be more than the kidneys can handle, the extra glucose spills out into the urine.

WHAT ARE THE DIFFERENT "TYPES" OF DIABETES?

As you already know, diabetes occurs in several forms. We used to think of the disorder as being "juvenile onset" and "maturity onset", but these terms really are not correct. We now prefer to call them insulin-dependent and noninsulin-dependent diabetes—or Type I and Type II.

Another type of diabetes is called "gestational" diabetes. It occurs only during pregnancy. Although gestational diabetes goes away after the baby is born, women who have had it are at higher risk for Type II diabetes later on.

Type II diabetes usually occurs after age 40—but not always. Similarly, Type I usually occurs in younger people, but as many as 15 to 20 percent are older when the disease develops.

An individual who has blood glucose levels above normal but not high enough to meet the present criterion for diagnosis of diabetes has "impaired glucose tolerance". It is especially important for these people to make changes in their eating habits and to lose weight if needed. Regular

blood glucose tests should be done by the doctor. This
condition can progress to Type II diabetes.

TYPES OF DIABETES

	Type I Insulin-Dependent	Type II Non-Insulin-Dependent
Who develops it?	Usually children or young adults	Usually overweight adults over age 40.
What is the cause?	Pancreas becomes unable to make insulin.	Body becomes unable to use insulin as it should.
How does a person feel?	Very thirsty, hungry and tired and needs to urinate often. May have stomach pain and become very ill if diabetes is not treated right away.	May not notice anything unusual, or may be tired and thirsty and need to urinate often.
What is done to control diabetes?	Healthy diet, exercise and daily insulin injections.	Healthy diet, exercise and sometimes diabetes pills or insulin injections.

ABOUT TYPE I DIABETES

With Type I diabetes, the insulin producing islet cells have
been destroyed. We don't know exactly how this happens.
Sometimes it seems the body's own immune system
destroys the cells, maybe because they seem abnormal. The
immune system normally protects us from germs or
infections attacking from outside our bodies. But sometimes
the system makes mistakes. Another theory is that certain
viruses may attack the beta cells and make them look
foreign to the body. The immune system then destroys the
beta cells.

Type I diabetes also is called "ketosis prone" diabetes. When
glucose can't be used for energy because no insulin is
present, the body will break down fat for energy. This

process releases more ketones into the blood than the body can handle. Ketones are acids, and if they build up, they can cause a serious condition called ketoacidosis.

Insulin injections are absolutely critical for people with Type I diabetes. They have no other choice.

AND TYPE II

In Type II diabetes, the pancreas usually looks normal. Beta cells still produce insulin. When scientists measure the insulin in the blood of people with Type II diabetes, the amounts usually are normal—and sometimes above normal. This puzzled everyone for a long time.

We now know a little more about how this works. On the walls of the cells are what are called "receptor sites." These are the keyholes that can be unlocked by insulin to allow glucose to enter the cell. With Type II diabetes, the number of receptor sites is low in some people. In others, the insulin simply doesn't seem to be able to stay "hooked". These people are "resistant" to their own insulin.

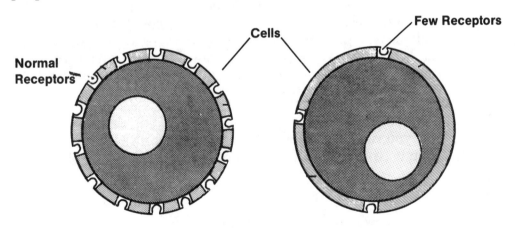

Being overweight can increase some people's resistance to insulin. One way of overcoming that resistance is losing weight and/or adding diabetes pills or adding extra insulin by injections. In many instances, losing weight allows the body to handle it's own insulin needs.

Heredity also plays a major role, since many people who are overweight don't develop diabetes. Sometimes the hereditary factor alone is enough to cause the insulin resistance and lead to diabetes. A combination of a hereditary tendency for Type II diabetes and extra weight most likely is involved in many individuals who develop diabetes. However, not all people with Type II diabetes are overweight.

People often ask if their Type II diabetes will eventually turn into Type I. This is a tricky question to answer.

As mentioned earlier, in some people with Type II, the beta cells may start to shut down—and the pancreas does not produce the total amount of insulin needed by the body to overcome insulin resistance and make up the deficit. Many of these individuals will need to take insulin by injection. Strictly speaking, however, this doesn't mean Type II diabetes is now Type I. Will it ever become Type I? It could. An individual with Type II diabetes who notices the classic symptoms of Type I (see the chart on page 10) **and** has ketones would be reclassified as having Type I diabetes.

The goal in managing your Type II diabetes is to keep your blood glucose levels as near normal as possible. The best advice is to put your treatment plan together and stick with it. Even if you do need insulin someday, don't give up on meal planning and exercise. And if your diabetes is newly diagnosed, we strongly encourage you to begin to take care of it right away.

As you read on, we hope we can give you the information you need to control your diabetes—so it won't control you.

CHAPTER 2

WHAT IS GOOD CONTROL AND HOW DO WE MEASURE IT?

We hear a lot about the importance of being in control of our lives. And yet that control can be fleeting. One moment things are going well, the next we are forced to relinquish control to forces beyond ourselves—whether they be storms, floods, fire or disease.

With Type II diabetes, we talk about control a lot—particularly control of blood glucose levels and of blood fats (cholesterol and triglyceride). We believe control is the key to a healthy way of living with diabetes. The tools are there for us to use, but we must decide to take charge and do what needs to be done.

WHAT DO WE MEAN BY "CONTROL"?

Blood Glucose Control

Everyone's blood glucose values vary throughout the day. Many factors influence this: food, exercise, medications, and stresses, to name a few. Good control means balancing these factors to keep glucoses as close to normal as possible.

It's difficult to say exactly what "normal" blood glucose is. For individuals who don't have diabetes, the blood glucose levels are almost always between 60 and 160 milligrams of glucose per deciliter of blood (mg/dl).

With diabetes, we need to look at the blood glucose before meals and one to two hours after meals to understand how you are doing. A comfortable goal before meals is 60 to 110 mg. After meals, aim for levels below 160 mg/dl.

Although it's ideal to have your blood glucose levels in these ranges, it may not be realistic. Ask your doctor or health care professional to help you find a goal or target that's right for you. And don't be disappointed if your blood glucose levels don't fall to where you want them right away.

Anything you can do to bring high levels down brings you a step closer to your personal goal.

Blood Fat Control
We know cholesterol and triglycerides are higher in persons whose blood glucose is elevated over a period of time. Measuring these is another way to "see how you are doing". They should be checked approximately once a year. Ideally cholesterol should be under 200 mg/dl and triglycerides under 150 mg/dl.

HOW DO YOU KNOW WHAT YOUR BLOOD GLUCOSE LEVEL IS?

The science of blood glucose monitoring has exploded during the last few years. You now can measure the amount of glucose in your blood by a simple test—at home, at work, in a restaurant, on an airplane, almost anywhere.

Monitoring involves getting a drop of blood from your finger and checking it by a chemically treated strip or with a meter. We'll tell you more about the specifics of monitoring in chapter 8.

In the past, and even now, some people use urine tests to determine blood glucose levels. We seldom recommend this because urine tests reflect only what the blood glucose level **has been** and that the blood glucose was elevated enough for the kidneys to begin filtering it out. It is possible for the blood glucose to be too high for good control without registering on a urine test strip.

Another test for people with diabetes is the hemoglobin A_1c or glycosylated hemoglobin. (Glycosylated hemoglobin means glucose attached to the hemoglobin portion of red blood cells. The more glucose the red blood cell has been exposed to, the more glucose will be attached to it.) This is a blood test that gives us a clue to overall control of blood glucose over a period of months. It must be done in a laboratory so your doctor must order it for you. Normal values will vary from laboratory to laboratory, based on the method used for performing the test. Usually it is done once every three or four months.

HIGH VS. LOW BLOOD GLUCOSE

Hyperglycemia—*hyper* meaning high, *glyc* meaning glucose, and *emia* meaning in the blood—is the technical name given to an elevated blood glucose level. Symptoms might include increased tiredness, thirst, or increased urination. As you already know, however, blood glucose can be very high without causing any obvious symptoms.

The opposite of hyperglycemia is hypoglycemia—with *hypo* meaning low. The term is used for blood glucose levels below 60 mg/dl. When blood glucose falls to low levels, you may have symptoms such as sweating, shaking, paleness, blurring vision, hunger, headache, dizziness or lightheadedness. This is the way your body signals you that it needs more glucose.

We emphasize control of blood glucose levels—and avoiding too many highs or too many lows—for your day-to-day and long term well being.

CHAPTER 3

EMOTIONS: THEY AFFECT US EVEN WHEN WE IGNORE THEM

When Jack Benny was being given a prestigious award some years ago, he accepted it with this comment: "Thanks, I really don't deserve this. But then, I have arthritis and I don't deserve that either." Jack might well have said diabetes instead of arthritis.

He lived a long and vigorous life with Type II diabetes—quite different from his own mother who died at age 47 with diabetes and cancer. According to the biography written by Jack's wife, Mary Livingston, Jack diagnosed his own diabetes. He was on a plane when he found an article about diabetes in *Readers' Digest*. He turned to his manager and said, "I have all these symptoms. I must have diabetes." Immediately after getting off the plane, he went to a doctor who confirmed the diagnosis. From then on, Jack did everything necessary to manage his diabetes.

What helps some people rise above their circumstances and move on with managing their lives, while others seem to struggle to stay in control? Part of the answer lies in how we deal with our feelings and how we talk to ourselves about what is happening.

FEELING OUR WAY

One of the toughest parts of learning you have a chronic disease is what that does to you emotionally. You may have all sorts of feelings—denial, fear, anger, guilt, depression.

These emotions are not unique to individuals or families with diabetes. Everyone feels them from time to time. They aren't good or bad, healthy or harmful. Each one can be helpful and useful to you as you work toward living well. But each also can become unhealthy and interfere with your life. Understanding how that can happen might help you recognize and avoid problems.

WHAT DETERMINES IF AN EMOTION IS HEALTHY OR UNHEALTHY?

An emotion becomes unhealthy when it upsets the balance you are striving for—that is, living well. For example, people who deny they have diabetes for long periods of time or who deny it is serious and permanent will manage their health poorly. An equally unhealthy balance will result if a person is extremely fearful and unnecessarily restricts activities.

Two factors largely determine whether an emotion will interfere in your life: its *intensity* or how strongly you feel it and its *duration*—how long you feel it.

Feeling is not an all-or-nothing process. You don't feel guilty about everything or about nothing. Instead, you have guilt within a range between those extremes. And you will likely feel different amounts of an emotion at different times.

You might feel very depressed at one point, mildly sad at another, and not at all depressed on a third occasion. When you do feel an emotion to an extreme degree—intense fear, for example—your ability to maintain the balance between living fully and managing diabetes is reduced.

How long you experience an emotion is also important. It's very normal and healthy for people to be angry when they learn they or a loved one has diabetes. However, if they continue to feel anger about the disease several years later, this is clearly unhealthy. It will interfere with the long-term management of diabetes.

Is there a time limit on how long an individual can feel an emotion before it becomes unhealthy? Is there an amount beyond which an emotion is too strong? No. Just as there isn't one right insulin dose or caloric intake for everyone, there isn't one right length of time or intensity to feel emotions.

Each of us responds differently, and it's important to recognize and accept those differences. Just as with food and insulin, though, extremes can be a problem.

WHAT ARE YOU FEELING?

We've all felt them, but do we really recognize them in ourselves? And do we understand them? They're the emotions most of us have when we learn about diabetes. Do you recognize any of the following?

DENIAL—DISBELIEF

"This isn't really happening."

"Come on, I'm not sick. I'll just wait a year or two and see what happens."

"It's not that serious."

"I don't have to feel anything about my diabetes."

It's natural to avoid unpleasant and scary feelings and to deny the reality of having diabetes. This disbelief can be healthy and protective at first. It insulates you from all the frightening, confusing feelings that would be overwhelming if you let them in all at once. It "buys time" for you to get used to your situation and the required changes.

We use denial every day. We don't believe that accidents, natural disasters, assaults, etc., will happen to us. Otherwise we would live in constant worry. However, denial is unhealthy when it affects how we take care of ourselves. If we believe we are specially protected and therefore don't need to wear seatbelts or quit smoking or stop abusing alcohol, we deny some very real risks. That's true with diabetes also.

If you deny your diabetes, you won't care for yourself as you should. You then suffer the consequences of feeling ill, lacking energy, and risking future health.

FEAR

"What will this mean for my life?"

"What's going to happen?"

As denial grows weaker, the reality of a situation becomes increasingly clear. You or your loved one has diabetes, and you are going to need to make some changes. But what does it all mean? Will you still be able to live a full life?

Diabetes is serious. It does require change—and that's frightening. It's common to feel you've lost control over your body; it has betrayed you by not functioning as it should. And you don't have enough information yet to regain control of your body and your life. You might feel anything from mild nervousness to downright terror, and the intensity of your fear may change from time to time.

Believe it or not, fear also has a purpose. It's fear, along with the discomfort of being out of control, that can motivate you to seek the answers you need to live well. Appropriate fear, which is really just respect for consequences or danger, motivates us to proceed carefully. On the other hand, too much fear over a long period of time can lead to hopelessness and the sense that it doesn't matter anyway.

If family members or others are too fearful about diabetes, they sometimes become overly protective. They may unnecessarily restrict activities or insist on strict management. Over time, this can lead to rebellion against those rigid demands and the person who makes them.

ANGER

"Why me?"

"It isn't fair!"

Everyone who has diabetes or loves someone who has diabetes feels angry at one time or another. It's a natural reaction to the unwanted, unexpected, undeserved and out of control situation we see ourselves in.

Anger, too, is healthy and normal. It can give us the energy we need to deal with or remove ourselves from unpleasant situations. You can't remove the diabetes. However, your anger can rally energy to help you deal with it. It's important to recognize your anger and accept that it's all right to be angry for a while.

Anger becomes unhealthy when it's felt too strongly for too long a period or is directed in a harmful manner. Sometimes we take the anger out on people around us—and sometimes we take it out on ourselves by not doing what needs to be done.

GUILT

"What did I do to deserve this?"

"If I just hadn't eaten so much sugar."

Guilt is an emotion we feel when we believe we are responsible for something bad happening. Some guilt is healthy and useful. We need to have a conscience to live responsibly. We sometimes need a little guilt to get us back on track—to stick to a meal plan or test blood glucose regularly. If you feel too guilty, though, you may give yourself messages that you are "bad" or a "failure."

These messages are likely to erode your self-esteem and make you less happy, less effective and less likely to take care of yourself.

SADNESS—DEPRESSION

"I feel so sad."

"I just don't feel like doing anything."

"I feel so alone. No one understands."

After you've tried a number of ways to cope with diabetes— you've avoided or denied it, you've been afraid and sought information, you've been angry—you realize diabetes will not go away, and you may feel depressed, sad, defeated, or resigned.

Sadness is a normal response to being unable to change situations we don't like. Diabetes and the changes it requires are forever. You can't make them go away.

Recognizing and accepting your sad feelings are important for your adjustment to diabetes. During the time you are sad, you often make the necessary changes in your self-image to include diabetes. This is a very important part of adjustment. It helps you focus on your new limits and the changes you must make. You learn to accept your new life, like many others before you.

We all have to accept limitations in life. Maybe we just can't be the tall, beautiful, athletic, artistic, rich people we always planned to be. That can make us sad, but usually we can accept who we are and move on.

Depression becomes unhealthy when it lasts too long and leads to loss of energy, decreased appetite, and sleeping problems. Self-imposed isolation can make us feel still more depressed and eventually can lead to feelings of hopelessness. When this happens, it becomes increasingly difficult to take care of ourselves.

ACCEPTANCE

"I don't always like watching how much food I eat, but I understand how important that is for me."

"I have diabetes, so I guess I'm going to have to make some changes."

For most of us, we come to the time when we *accept* our diabetes. This doesn't mean we like it, want it, or feel happy about it. It just means we admit to ourselves and others that we have diabetes. It's part of us.

At this point, we can choose to make the needed changes good management requires. But at the same time, we can avoid setting unnecessary limits or restrictions. We can balance. Once we accept, we can focus on strengths instead of limitations.

Does everyone experience the same process of adjustment in order to reach acceptance?

While most people have many of the feelings we've talked about, each of us is unique. Our emotional responses also are unique. Adjustment is not a neat, orderly, predictable process we all move through the same way. We don't move from one feeling to another and then magically reach acceptance and live happily ever after.

Is acceptance forever? Not exactly. Just as a smooth pond will ripple now and then, your acceptance will ripple also. Sometimes the long-term, "forever" aspect of diabetes will just be too much. Or other events in life will trigger the old fears or anger or sadness about diabetes. It isn't unusual to have old feelings return. In fact, sometimes you might go through the whole process, again reaching acceptance.

Other feelings often come with acceptance. Feelings such as pride. You can feel proud of yourself—proud you are coping well, taking excellent care of yourself, meeting your challenges. You feel in control of your diabetes and your life. You are the driver rather than the helpless bystander. You can feel hope, not necessarily that a cure for diabetes will be found tomorrow, but that the growing knowledge and understanding of the disease will help you live fully and well with diabetes.

We suspect you have felt, or may feel, all of these emotions at some time or another. Please remember the feelings are normal and healthy. But if you get stuck on any one of them for too long or if you see someone you love struggling to overcome some of these feelings, they may become a problem.

HOW DO YOU KNOW WHEN YOUR EMOTIONS BECOME A PROBLEM?

If you are aware of the balance you want to maintain, then you can be aware when that balance is tipped. If your diabetes is out of control or if there is a problem area within the rest of your life—conflict within your family, difficulties at work, problems with friends, or limitations in your activities—it's time to ask yourself some questions.

Why are you experiencing this difficulty? If your diabetes is out of control, have you changed medication, food, or activities. Is this a long-term problem? Problems in the rest of your life will not always be related to your diabetes. For example, you may simply be having difficulty with a work project or dislike your new boss. However, there are also times when your feelings about diabetes will affect how you interact with family members, friends, and employers, and which activities you choose to participate in or limit.

What can you do once you determine some of your feelings have become an obstacle to living well with diabetes:

Identifying that there is a problem is a healthy, positive first step. Next you must try to identify what you are feeling.

Often when you know what you are feeling, you can change how you express this feeling. For example, once you know you are really angry at your diabetes and not at your spouse, you can work toward expressing anger in a way that won't hurt you or others.

You might release this anger through sports or exercise, or talk it out with family members, friends, or clergy. If you recognize it's fear that stops you from becoming independent or guilt that keeps you from setting limits, you might be able to take a deep breath and let go—a little at a time—or feel better about setting some realistic expectations.

These changes may not be easy, and they won't happen overnight. You can change what you feel and how you express your emotions. Sometimes you might need help.

It's often hard to struggle with feelings alone. Support from others can be critical. You need to accept and actively seek emotional support from family, friends, and your health care team. Some people find it very rewarding to join a support group made up of others experiencing similar feelings or challenges. Contact your local chapter of the American Diabetes Association for information about support groups in your area.

If you have identified a problem related to your feelings about diabetes and have struggled with this problem alone or talked with family and friends and realize it's something you need help with, it's time to seek professional help. Counselors, social workers, and psychologists are skilled in guiding you in identifying feelings and working toward a healthy expression of them. This could be a key to successfully coping with diabetes in oneself or a family member. The earlier this action is taken, the easier it will be to work out a solution.

HERE ARE SOME CLUES TO HELP YOU IDENTIFY WHAT YOU MAY BE FEELING:

- Do you feel that you can avoid taking care of your diabetes without consequences?
- Do you hope that if you ignore your diabetes it will somehow go away?
- Do you feel that you are no different now than you were before you developed diabetes, and that *you don't need to change?*

  If so, you may be feeling disbelief, denying that you truly have diabetes, that it is permanent, that it is serious, or that it's going to take time to adjust to.

- Are you absolutely rigid about your meal plan and medication times?
- Do you feel that diabetes has so many possible complications that your situation is hopeless?

  If so, you may be feeling fear.

- Do you feel life is terribly unfair?
- Do you find yourself irritable with family members, friends, or health care team members for no apparent reason?
- Do you refuse to follow the recommendations of your health care team?

  Perhaps you are angry.

- Do you expect less of your family member with diabetes because he or she already has enough to deal with?
- Do you feel like a failure when even one blood glucose test is high?

  Then you may be experiencing guilt.

- Do you feel no one else can understand what you're going through?
- Do you feel hopeless?
- Do you find yourself teary-eyed frequently?

  Then you may be experiencing sadness or depression.

CHAPTER 4

NUTRITION: FUELING UP FOR BETTER HEALTH

Many people think having diabetes means you can't eat sugar. That's partially correct. True, sugars and starches cause blood glucose to rise, but so do all foods—meats, dairy products, fruits, or juices. So in fact, you need to limit portions of all foods.

You may be wondering what you can eat—or wondering if you need to cook separate meals for yourself and your family, etc. These are valid concerns. There is help available to you. Ask your doctor to refer you to a registered dietitian (a health professional with the letters R.D. after her or his name) or a diabetes nutrition specialist. Dietitians can answer these and other questions for you. They can prepare a meal plan for you and advise you of foods to choose, what to look for when you go grocery shopping, how to prepare foods in a healthy way for you and your family, and much more.

Fortunately the meal plan we want you to follow is the same one we suggest for all Americans. The following guidelines are the basis for the nutrition recommendations we make.

1. Lighten Up!

It's important for all of us to work toward a reasonable body weight by increasing our physical activities and cutting back on the amount of food we eat. In general, weight loss improves blood pressure and blood fat (cholesterol and triglyceride) levels. In people with diabetes, losing weight can improve blood glucose levels.

The following occurs with weight loss:

Weight loss
↓
Body cells become sensitive to insulin
↓
Cells use glucose
↓
Blood glucose levels begin to return to normal

How much weight must a person lose to see these effects? Often surprisingly little, Improvement in glucose levels can happen with a small to moderate loss (5-15 pounds).

2. Team Up With Carbohydrates.

Eat more starches, fiber, and naturally occurring sugars. Use fewer refined and processed sugars.

There are different kinds of carbohydrates:

- Starches or complex carbohydrates
  This group includes starchy vegetables and grain and cereal products such as breads, potatoes, corn, peas, cereals, pasta, rice, etc.

- Sugar
  There are two major forms of sugar:
  naturally occurring sugars—such as those found in fruits, vegetables, and milk
  refined or processed sugars—such as table sugars, honey, jam, jelly, syrups soda pop, pies, cakes and icings, etc.

- Fiber
  This is the indigestible carbohydrate portion of foods which adds bulk to our diets. This group includes fruits, vegetables, grains and cereal products. (Dairy products, meats and fats do not contain fiber.)

The goal is to avoid as many of the refined sugars and sweets as possible and use more foods containing starch (complex carbohydrate), fiber and naturally occurring sugars.

Contrary to popular belief, starches often have fewer calories than foods with large amounts of fat and sugar. Starches indeed are very good for us!

3. Trim fat. Lean toward lean.

Reduce the amount of fat and cholesterol in your diet (especially saturated fat). To do this choose foods low in fat and cholesterol. (More about fats on page 41).

Not only is fat high in calories, but a diet high in fat also greatly increases our risk for heart disease and heart attacks. All Americans are at risk for heart disease, but the risk is greater for persons with diabetes.

4. Shake the salt habit.

Limit salt in cooking, do not add salt to foods at the table, and avoid salty snacks. Choose more fresh foods and fewer processed and fast foods. (More about reducing salt in diet on page 46.)

A diet high in salt, obesity and an inherited tendency increase the risk of developing high blood pressure. People with diabetes are at a greater risk for developing high blood pressure. So it is important to reduce as many of the risk factors as possible.

5. Emphasize variety.

"Variety is the spice of life." This is a good way to be sure that you will not have too much or too little of any of the vitamins or minerals your body needs. A variety of foods contributes to good health—and to good taste.

These dietary goals apply to all persons—whether or not they have diabetes.

WHEN YOU HAVE DIABETES

One additional goal for individuals with diabetes is to avoid high blood glucose and blood fat levels and the possible consequences of them. In other words, control diabetes.

Following the dietary goals is a good start. Equally important as what you eat is when and how much you eat. Spacing meals throughout the day and eating smaller amounts of food at each meal help improve glucose levels.

• **When you eat.** Regularly spaced meals (breakfast, lunch, dinner, and possibly some snacks) will allow your body the time needed to bring blood glucoses down before the next meal.

After eating, food is digested and much of it goes into the blood stream as glucose (blood glucose). It stays there until it is taken into the cell where it is used for energy. As the glucose enters the cell the blood levels go down. How fast it goes down depends in part on how efficient your body's insulin is.

Eating large meals during the day gives your body a very large amount of food to use at one time. More food will result in more glucose. Your body may not be able to respond with enough effective insulin to bring the blood glucose down. You are in effect, taxing an already inefficient system.

Spaced meals help control your blood glucose and appetite, while giving your body energy when you need it—during the day when you are most active.

• **What and how much you eat.** What and how much you eat not only affects your weight, but also your blood glucoses day-to-day, meal-to-meal. By monitoring your blood glucoses, you will begin to see what happens when you eat a larger than usual meal or snack. You will begin to know what happens when you delay or skip meals. (By the way, we don't recommend you do that!)

Take a moment to think about your eating habits and these dietary goals. What habits should you keep? What changes can you make?

How do you rate yourself on the following?

	Usually Not	Occasionally (How often or how much?)	Frequently (How often or how much?)
Spaced meals			
Regular meal times			
Use refined and processed sugars (pop, syrup, desserts, sweets)			
Meat portions: More than 4 oz. per serving			
Use high fat meats (lunch meats, bacon, sausage, prime meats)			
Fats Butter/margarine			
Salad dressings			
Sauces/gravies			
Starches: Avoid most because they are fattening or cause blood glucose to rise			
Salt: Use at table			
Add as cooking foods			
Use convenience foods			
Use processed meats			

HOW DO YOU DO IT?

You know what you eat. Now you have some idea of what we recommend.

There really is no magic involved in coming up with a meal plan. You will want to have a meal plan that is the right number of calories for you considering your level of activity, your age and whether or not you need to lose weight. After you know how many calories you need to reach your weight goal, you are ready to decide what foods you will eat and to set the portion sizes. This will be your meal plan.

Let's go through it step-by-step.

HOW MANY CALORIES DO YOU NEED?

First, you need to determine your desirable body weight (DBW) using this formula:

Women: 100 pounds for the first five feet
5 pounds for each additional inch

Men: 106 pounds for the first five feet
6 pounds for each additional inch

Add 10% for a large body frame; subtract 10% for a small body frame.

Remember, this is a desirable body weight—not necessarily your weight goal. This is the number we use to decide how many calories our bodies need each day. Most of us are going to think these weights are terribly low. The important thing is to start moving in the right direction.

Here's an example of how to find your desirable body weight.

Mary is 5'6" tall, and her frame is average; her desirable body weight is 130.

$$
\begin{array}{r}
100 \text{ lbs} \\
+ \ \underline{30 \text{ lbs}} \quad (6 \text{ inches x 5 lbs per inch}) \\
130 \text{ lbs}
\end{array}
$$

Figure your desirable body weight and record it here.

_____

Next determine the number of calories you need to maintain your DBW.

Choose the number that best fits your activity level.

- 15 calories per pound of DBW for active men or very active women.

- 13 calories per pound of DBW for active women and sedentary men and individuals over age 55.

- 10 calories per pound of DBW for sedentary very obese individuals or chronic dieters.

Example: Bob is 57 years old. His DBW is 173 pounds and he is active. Because he is over 55, he uses 13 calories per pound as his guide. He needs 2250 calories per day to maintain his DBW.

$$173 \times 13 = 2249 \ (2250)$$

Figure your daily calorie requirement and record it here.

_____ DBW

x _____ Calories per pound

= _____ Daily calorie requirement

Now, to lose weight you must burn more fuel (measured in calories) than you eat. One pound of body fat contains approximately 3500 calories.

To lose one pound, you will need to eat 3500 fewer calories or increase your activity to burn more of the calories you eat. Cut down 500 calories per day from your daily calorie needs to lose a pound per week.

Bob, in the example above, needs 1750 calories per day to lose one pound of fat per week.

$$2250 - 500 = 1750$$

Figure your daily caloric requirement to lose weight.

_____ Calorie requirement

- _____ Less the calories to lose weight

= _____ Weight loss requirement

The lowest number of calories recommended for women is 1200 calories per day. Men need a minimum of 1500 calories per day. To lose weight faster than one pound per week without the danger of eating too few calories, increase the amount of exercise you do. This allows you to eat adequate amounts of food and still lose weight.

WHAT CAN I EAT?

Once you know how many calories you need, the next step is to decide what and how much food to eat for meals and snacks. One way to do this is to set up a meal plan using the "exchange" system.

In the exchange system similar foods are grouped together. (You can use the word "serving" instead of "exchange".) Each group (there are six of these) includes foods that are similar in carbohydrate, protein, fat, and calories when you choose them in the amounts listed.

When your meal plan lists the number of servings or exchanges from a food group, you can choose from any of the foods in that group. The portion size or serving of the food will also be listed.

Your meal plan tells you how many servings to choose from each group for your meals and snacks. It is like a "budget" that guides you in "spending" the calories for each day.

For example, if you plan 2 starch exchanges at breakfast, you might choose 1 slice of toast and 1/2 cup of hot cereal, or you might choose 1 cup of hot cereal (2 starch exchanges) and no toast. You could also choose 2 English muffin halves (2 starch exchanges) and no cereal.

When setting up your meal plan, use this general calorie guide. It lists the portion size and the approximate number of calories for foods in each group. For more detail, use Exchange Lists for Meal Planning.

Calorie Content Guide

Food Group	Serving Size	Calories
1. Starch/bread	1 slice bread, 1/2 cup pasta, starchy vegetable, potato, 1/2 to 3/4 cup cereal, 4 or 6 crackers	80
2. Meat and substitute	1 oz. cooked lean meat (poulty, fish, lean beef, canned ham) 1/4 cup cottage cheese	55
	1 oz. cooked medium fat meat (beef or pork roast, steak, lean ground beef), liver, 1 egg	75
3. Vegetable (non-starchy)	1/2 cup cooked, 1 cup raw	25
4. Fruit	1/2 cup canned or frozen without sugar, 1 medium serving of fresh, 1 cup melon or berries, 1/4 cup dried fruit	60
5. Milk	8 oz. skim or low-fat milk 8 oz. plain low-fat yogurt	90
6. Fat	1 teaspoon margarine, oil or mayonnaise 1 tablespoon salad dressing (French or Italian)	45

FIGURING YOUR MEAL PLAN

• Two servings from each group provide your basic nutrition needs.

• Decide how many servings from each group you want during the day.

• Record your choices on the form below.

• Multiply the number of servings by the calories per serving to determine the total calories from each food group. Record these numbers.

• Add together all the numbers in the calorie column to arrive at the total calories. Record this number.

• If you are not satisfied with your total number of calories, go back over your choices and make changes.

Food Group	No. of servings that you desire	Calories per serving	Calories
1. Starch/bread	_____	x 80 =	_____
2. Meat and substitute	_____	x 75 =	_____
3. Vegetable	_____	x 25 =	_____
4. Fruit	_____	x 60 =	_____
5. Milk, skim	_____	x 90 =	_____
6. Fat	_____	x 45 =	_____
		Total Calories	_____

To see how close your meal plan comes to fitting the recommendations outlined earlier in this chapter, your dietitian can figure out how many of your calories come from carbohydrate, protein and fat and the percentage of calories from each.

	Typical American diet	Recommended diet
Carbohydrate	30-40%	50-60%
Protein	12-18%	12-18%
Fat	40-50%	25-30%

Your Plan:

	Grams	Calories	Percent
Carbohydrate			
Protein			
Fat			
Total Calories			

After deciding the number of servings from each group that you want on your plan and arriving at the correct calorie level, divide these servings into meals and snacks for the day.

Your meal plan	Sample menu

Breakfast

_____ Starch _____
_____ Meat _____
_____ Fruit _____
_____ Milk _____
_____ Fat _____

Morning snack

_____ _____
_____ _____
_____ _____

Lunch

_____ Starch _____
_____ Meat _____
_____ Vegetable _____
_____ Fruit _____
_____ Milk _____
_____ Fat _____

Afternoon snack

_____ _____
_____ _____
_____ _____

Dinner

_____ Starch _____
_____ Meat _____
_____ Vegetable _____
_____ Fruit _____
_____ Milk _____
_____ Fat _____

Bedtime snack

_____ _____
_____ _____
_____ _____

There is no one right meal plan. Consider your personal preferences and apply the general guidelines of spaced, regular meals, low in fat, high in starch (complex carbohydrate) and low in refined sugars. Some people like large breakfasts, others don't. Some like a mid-afternoon snack because they have a late supper. Others like to have an early supper. You are the one who decides what you eat and when you eat it.

If a meal plan doesn't fit your lifestyle, you probably won't follow it. So do build your meal plan around your needs.

Note: If you are on insulin, you may need snacks at specific times. Be sure to follow your health professionals guidance about your specific concerns.

CHAPTER 5

TIPS FOR CHOOSING FOODS

WHAT YOU NEED TO KNOW ABOUT FAT

Somewhere along the way, someone must have decided the word "fat" was inelegant. So a fancier name was adopted. LIPIDS.

You probably won't hear too much about fat in your blood, but you might hear about blood lipids. Don't be confused. Lipids are fats.

We're beginning to understand how important lipid levels are for good health.

Blood lipids come in several varieties: cholesterol, HDL—cholesterol, LDL—cholesterol, and triglycerides. Here are some definitions that might help you sort out the differences.

Cholesterol: a fat-like waxy substance made by the body and present only in animal foods. A certain amount is needed for many of our body's chemical processes. Too much, however, increases the risk of heart disease. To reach a healthy cholesterol level (less than 200 milligrams), eat fewer foods high in cholesterol and saturated fats.

Cholesterol is carried through our blood stream by lipoproteins. Two major carriers of cholesterol are LDL and HDL.

LDL—Cholesterol: "LDL" means low-density lipoprotein. This is another carrier of cholesterol. It is referred to as the "bad" cholesterol. It is linked to major problems with the blood vessels and heart.

HDL—Cholesterol: "HDL" stands for high-density lipoprotein. It is one of the carriers of cholesterol in the blood stream. This is sometimes referred to as the "good" cholesterol. It protects against heart disease and actually removes fat from blood vessels. This cholesterol is not affected by diet but is increased by regular exercise.

Triglycerides: The form in which fat is found in most foods. Also the form in which fat is carried in the blood stream and stored in fat cells. When we take in a lot of calories, triglyceride levels tend to go up. Also, high blood glucose levels can lead to high triglyceride levels in the blood. Alcohol tends to raise the triglycerides in the blood quickly, as does eating large amounts of concentrated sweets.

A NOTE ABOUT FOOD FATS

Now, at the risk of really confusing you, we'll tell you the fat we eat comes in several varieties as well. There's saturated, polyunsaturated, and mono-unsaturated fat, plus omega-3 fatty acids.

Saturated fats: They usually are solid at room temperature. Large amounts of saturated fats are the major cause of high blood cholesterol levels. It's best to avoid these whenever possible.

Most saturated fats come from animal sources (lard, butter and butterfat-containing dairy products, meats), but a few are from plants. Saturated plant fats are palm and coconut oil, cocoa butter, and solid shortenings made from vegetable fats.

Polyunsaturated fats: These usually are from vegetables and are liquid at room temperature. These fats can help lower blood cholesterol, although we don't know exactly how or why. Polyunsaturated fats include safflower, corn, sunflower, soybean and cottonseed oils and walnuts. These fats are better choices than saturated fats.

Mono-unsaturated fats: At one time we thought these fats were neutral—that they neither raised nor lowered cholesterol levels. Recently we've learned these fats lower "bad" cholesterol levels but do not affect "good" levels. Fats in this group are olive oil, peanut oil, nuts (except walnuts) and olives.

Omega-3 fatty acids: These oils are found in cold water and "fatty" fish. They lower triglycerides and cholesterol and decrease the clotting of blood. Some good sources of omega-3 fatty acids are salmon, tuna, mackerel, herring, trout, crab, shrimp, lobster, and cod. You may have heard about the fish oil supplements that contain these oils. It is not recommended that persons with diabetes use the supplements but instead eat fish 2 or 3 times a week.

REDUCING SATURATED FATS AND CHOLESTEROL IN YOUR DIET.

Here are some tips to help you cut down on fats.

1. Reduce portion sizes of meats (6 ounces or less daily). Select the leanest cuts of meats and remove all visible fat before eating. Use lean red meats, poultry (remove the skin), fish and vegetarian fare to replace high fat meats whenever possible.

2. Use low fat cooking methods: baking, broiling, roasting, grilling, or boiling foods—avoid frying. (Frying and breading add to the fat content and calories of the food.)

3. Skim fat from broths, soups, and gravies.

4. Limit use of high fat meats to 3 servings or less a week. This includes luncheon meats, cold cuts, salami, frankfurters, sausage, bacon, prime cuts of meats, rib or club steaks, spare ribs, canned meats (Spam, Treat, Stews, Chili).

5. Use low-fat and non-fat dairy products such as skim or 1% milk, plain low-fat yogurt and part skim milk cheeses. Limit or avoid dairy products containing large amounts of butterfat such as butter, whole milk, whole milk cheeses, ice cream, sour or sweet cream, cream cheese, etc.

6. Use margarine instead of butter. Choose one listing a liquid oil as the first ingredient on the label.

7. Limit use of commercial baked goods, processed foods, and fast foods.

8. Use vegetable oils in place of solid shortenings or butter whenever possible in baking or cooking and in salad dressings.

9. Limit egg yolks to three or less per week.

TRY SOME ALTERNATIVES:

1. Low-fat cottage cheese (2%) or no-fat cottage cheese.

2. Low-cholesterol cheeses (Cheezola, Taystee, Lite-Line, etc.). *These may not be low in salt.

3. Cheese made from skim milk (Mozzarella, Neufchatel, Farmer's Ricotta, Monterey Jack).

4. Commercially packaged thinly sliced lean beef, chicken, turkey, ham, luncheon meat labeled 95% fat free or turkey pastrami. (Not all of these will be low in salt.)

5. Low-cholesterol egg substitutes (Eggbeaters, Second Nature, Chono).

6. Two egg whites in place of one whole egg.

7. Instant nonfat dry milk powder in coffee instead of nondairy coffee creamers made with palm or coconut oil.

8. Low-fat yogurt as a base for creamy salad dressings and in place of sweet or sour cream.

9. In mayonnaise dressing recipes, replace some or all of the mayonnaise (100 calories/tablespoon) with plain low-fat yogurt (8 calories/tablespoon).

10. Party dip can be made by adding spices and flavorings to plain yogurt or blending low-fat cottage cheese, and adding lemon juice and herbs to taste.

11. Fruits as desserts or snacks.

12. More grains and grain products in your meal plan.

REDUCING SODIUM (SALT) IN YOUR DIET

As mentioned in the nutritional recommendations section, weight loss and reducing sodium in the diet are crucial for controlling blood pressure.

Table salt is a common source of sodium. (Table salt is approximately half sodium; the other part is chloride.) Sodium is the mineral that aggravates blood pressure.

The recommended amount of sodium per day is 2300 mg. the amount of sodium in 1 teaspoon of salt.

Salt = Sodium + Chloride

1 Teaspoon = 2300 mg. sodium

Reducing salt in your diet.

1. Use the salt shaker less often, if at all. Don't set it on the table.

2. Cook with less salt.

3. Limit your use of commercial snack goods, "convenience" processed foods, and fast foods. (Home-cooked is still best.)

4. Read package labels. The amount of sodium will be listed on product labels that carry nutritional labeling.

5. Carefully choose your condiments. High salt condiments include soy sauce, steak sauce, catsup, and seasoned salts.

6. These seasonings contain sodium and are best limited or avoided.

AVOID . . . Celery salt
Meat/vegetable extracts

Seasoned salt
Meat tenderizers

Garlic salt/Onion salt
Commercial bouillon (cubes or granules)

Cooking wine
Catsup

Chili sauce
Prepared mustard

Steak sauce
Table or seasoned salt

Barbecue sauce
Olives, pickles

Soy sauce
Monosodium glutamate

Worcestershire sauce
Brine

TRY SOME ALTERNATIVES:

1. Experiment with herbs and spices. Numerous salt free spice blends are available on the market, or make your own combinations.

2. A squeeze of lemon—lemon "bites" your tongue like salt.

3. Use fresh meats, fish, and poultry in place of luncheon meats, hot dogs, sausage, etc.

4. Reduce or omit (depending upon product) the amount of salt used in baking. (Experiment with the recipes).

5. Use onion **powder** and garlic **powder** in place of the "salts".

6. For snacks, choose fresh fruits or vegetables, unsalted nuts, or unsalted popcorn.

7. Rinse canned foods with fresh water to reduce the amount of sodium.

ADDING FIBER

Fiber is the parts of plant foods that are not broken down or digested in our bodies. "Roughage" is another term often used. It is found in the structural part of plants—the skin, roots, stems, leaves and seeds.

There are some major benefits of using more fiber in our diets. These include:

• A full and satisfied feeling that helps to control our appetites and helps with weight loss.

• High fiber foods many times are lower in calories, another benefit for those losing weight or keeping it off.

• Bowel regularity is improved. In addition to feeling more comfortable, the risks of colon cancer may be reduced.

• Certain types of fiber, especially that found in oat bran, some fruits such as apples and oranges and dry beans, peas and legumes, slow down how fast glucose is absorbed in the body. This type of fiber may have an effect on lowering blood glucose levels.

• Yet another benefit may be a decrease in blood cholesterol and triglycerides, the blood fats that increase risks for heart disease.

How much fiber should we eat? Most people get 10 to 15 grams per day. We recommend increasing this to 25 to 40 grams per day.

To get more fiber use whole grains, cereals and breads, vegetables, dried peas and beans and fruits. (There is no fiber in dairy products, meats, fish, poultry or fats.)

SOURCES OF FIBER

		Grams of fiber per serving
Cereals:	Oatmeal, Wheaties, Shredded Wheat, Bran Flakes, Grapenuts, Corn Bran, Chex (average 1/2 cup)	3
	100% Bran, All Bran, Bran Buds, Fiber One (1/3 - 1/2 cup)	8
Starchy Vegetables and Grains:	Corn, potatoes, brown rice, bulgur, peas (1/3 - 1/2 cup)	3
Dried Beans and Peas, Lentils	(1/3 cup)	4-5
Breads:	Whole grain breads and crackers (1 slice or 1 oz.)	2
Vegetables:	Raw or Cooked 1/2 - 3/4 cup cooked 1 - 2 cups raw	 2 3
Fruits:	Fresh or canned or frozen 1/2 cup or one medium fresh Dried fruits, 1/4 cup	 2 3

EATING AWAY FROM HOME

More people are eating away from home for its convenience during or after a long work day or while traveling. Whatever the reason for eating out, take those skills you've been practicing at home out with you. Keep in mind every food you eat is your choice. Use common sense when choosing and ENJOY yourself.

Know your meal plan and make the best choices from the menu. It may be helpful to carry a copy of your meal plan with you. (Write it on a small card and put it in your wallet.)

Watch portion sizes. Is it a bargain to get large portions when you eat out? It may not be if you eat all that is on your plate and that is more than what is on your meal plan. Practice measuring and weighing foods at home so you will recognize correct portion sizes when you are out. Portions too large? Take it home in a "people" bag.

Choose your eating out environment. The restaurant atmosphere will greatly influence your eating choices and behavior. Is it a fast food, fast service place: get you seated, served and out or is it a place that fosters slow dining, lingering and enjoying your meal so despite smaller portions you'll leave feeling satisfied?

Choose restaurants that offer a variety of foods that fit into your meal plan and budget. Unsure about what is served at a particular restaurant? Call ahead and ask! Ask the waitperson about particular foods and preparation if you are in doubt. When you place your order, be specific about what you want and how you want to have it served, such as dressing on the side, whole wheat bread for the sandwich, dry toast, plain baked potato with margarine on the side, etc.

Be on the lookout for fats. By planning ahead, you can move as many fat exchanges as you can spare from another time of the day to your meal out. (Meals out often contain more fats than meals prepared at home). Be aware that cooking methods can add unplanned for fats. Gravies and sauces also may contain fat. (Ask for them on the side if you use them at all.)

Avoid foods and beverages obviously high in sugar and fats. Some examples to avoid would include syrups, jams, most desserts, regular pop, gelatins, canned fruits, salad dressings, sauces, gravies. (Ask for low calorie dressings, syrups, jam.)

Think about timing of meals. Particularly if you take a diabetes medication, having your meals on time is critical for preventing hypoglycemia. Will your meal be delayed more than an hour? Have a fruit or starch exchange while you wait.

Did you blow it? There is one thing you can do: exercise. Granted it takes a lot of exercise to burn calories, but it helps. How about dancing or a brisk walk or a few miles on the exercise bike?

The next meal—get back to the plan.

In summary, don't leave everything you've learned about healthy eating choices at home. It's the same you in dress clothes or casual clothes. All the skills you've learned are portable. Tuck them into your pocket on your way out.

CAN YOU USE ALCOHOLIC BEVERAGES?

The answer depends upon several considerations, such as diabetes control, other medical conditions, other medications you might be taking, and what and how often you choose to drink.

• Avoid alcohol if your diabetes control is poor. Get your blood glucoses back into a better range. When diabetes is well controlled the blood glucoses are not greatly affected by the occasional use of alcohol.

• Avoid alcohol if you have any of these conditions:

High triglycerides: Drinking alcoholic beverages can raise the blood fat level and further increase the risk of heart disease.

Gastritis, pancreatitis, certain types of kidney and heart diseases: If you have any of these conditions, discuss alcohol use with your physician.

Diabetes pills and alcohol may not mix: Alcohol may react with some of the first generation diabetes pills to cause some unpleasant side effects. These include flushing or "becoming beet red", a rapid heart rate, dizziness, and nausea. When this occurs, stop drinking. This reaction is less likely to happen with the second generation diabetes pills.

Other medications: Always check with your physician or pharmacist whenever you start a medication to find out if alcohol can be used with it.

Can you afford the calories in alcohol? Alcohol contains a large number of empty calories and no other nutrients. Alcohol calories are usually converted to fat in our bodies and these extra calories make weight loss more difficult. Many drinks average 100 to 300 calories each.

Do not drink on an empty stomach. Alcohol can cause a lowering of blood glucose levels if you haven't eaten for several hours. So your risk for hypoglycemia is greater.

Remember, too, alcohol can impair your judgement. Don't let it make you careless with your meal plan.

GUIDELINES

- Limit your use to one or two drinks.
- Use alcohol no more than two times a week.
- Have with food.

Choose your mix	Amount	Watch the exchanges	Count the calories
Diet pop	Any amount	Free	0
Mineral Water	Any amount	Free	0
Diet tonic	Any amount	Free	0
Club soda	Any amount	Free	0
Juices			
Vegetable	1/2 cup	1 vegetable	25-35
Fruit	1/2 cup	1 fruit	60-80
Beer			
Light (preferred)	12 ounces	2 fat	100
Regular	12 ounces	1 starch, 2 fat	150
Liquor			
(any kind, 86 proof)	1 1/2 ounces	2 fat	80-100
Wine, dry	4 ounces	2 fat	75-100

CHAPTER 6

CHANGING EATING HABITS—
FOR THE BETTER

Andy Rooney sums up our feelings pretty well when he says: "The two biggest sellers in any bookstore are the cookbooks and the diet books. The cookbooks tell you how to prepare the food, and the diet books tell you how not to eat any of it."

Being overweight certainly is a major concern of our times. And with diabetes, too much weight is a cause for concern. We need to look at why we gain weight and what we can do to change the patterns we've developed.

It's important to remember that we've all developed habits over our lifetime, and we can't expect to change them overnight.

The goal is to eliminate habits that have contributed to your becoming overweight and replace them with habits more suited to losing weight and keeping it off. Again, this will be a gradual process of unlearning reactions to food that have been learned over a lifetime. But with effort and perserverance you can change habits.

BECOME AWARE OF YOUR
EATING HABITS AND MAKE
SPECIFIC PLANS TO CHANGE

There are three major strategies to use in changing eating patterns. The first strategy is to become aware of your eating habits.

Although you may feel you know all about your eating behavior, it is indeed rare to find someone who is aware of all of his/her eating patterns and what influences them. To become aware of your eating habits, keep a record of your food and beverage intake.

1. Record everything you eat and drink except water.
2. Record how long it takes to eat each meal and snack.
3. Record where you are eating and with whom.
4. Record what else you were doing while eating.
5. Record how hungry you were.

FOOD RECORD					
Time Start/Stop	Food and Amount	Where eaten?	With whom?	Doing what else?	How hungry?

If you keep records honestly for a week or two, you will discover things about yourself that you never before realized. As you review your records, you will see patterns. And you will no longer be able to fool yourself into thinking you have eaten less than you actually have. This self monitoring will develop the awareness, skills and attitudes that will be the foundation of any change you make in your eating habits.

Many behavior changes begin when you simply become more aware of what you are doing. For example, eating more slowly while sitting down and not doing other things while you are eating will keep you aware of the eating process. Continue to keep records throughout the behavior change process.

LOOK FOR WAYS TO AVOID SITUATIONS IN WHICH PROBLEM EATING OCCURS

The second strategy is to find ways to avoid situations in which problem eating occurs. People in our society usually do not eat because of physical hunger but because certain times, places and even people become associated with food and eating.

For example, if you are accustomed to reading the newspaper in the kitchen and nibbling because food is close at hand, you may have to find a different place to read the newspaper. Keeping food out of sight keeps it out of mind. It helps to keep food out of rooms other than the kitchen. Limit eating to one specific place in your home. Change your route if a particular store or vending machine is a problem. Clear the table immediately after eating.

LEARN TO RESPOND DIFFERENTLY TO SITUATIONS THAT CAUSE EATING PROBLEMS

While it is best to avoid problem eating situations, it is not always possible to do so. In this case a third strategy can be used. It is to plan out and learn to change how you respond to difficult eating situations.

For example, grocery shopping may be a necessity for you, but shopping on a full stomach and with a firm shopping list can reduce the chances of impulse buying. Planning daily menus helps reduce indecision at meal times.

Pre-planning can also reduce the tendency to overeat at parties or restaurants. Do not go without food all day so that you can eat as much as you want at a party. You will be so hungry when you arrive that you will eat far more than you should or want to. By avoiding long times without food you can arrive in a frame of mind to enjoy yourself but stick to your meal plan.

Try leaving a bit of food on your plate, and practice responding politely but firmly to people who try to encourage you to eat more than you intend.

BEING IN CHARGE

Many people say they don't have enough willpower to follow their meal plans. Our response to that is, "Don't count on willpower alone!" Rather plan how you can be in charge.

Also in the process of changing eating habits, remember that perfection is not demanded. Most diets are followed in the all-or-nothing fashion; you are either on the diet or off it. To expect such perfection is to set yourself up for failure.

No one is ever totally in control or out of control. By allowing yourself some leeway and looking for gradual and permanent changes, you will avoid the pitfalls of "dieting." Set realistic goals for yourself and view your weight loss as a series of small accomplishments, each one an important step toward the results you want for yourself.

The following specific tips have helped others like you make permanent changes in eating habits and lose weight:

1. **Slow down your eating speed.** By eating more slowly, you are less likely to finish off a second helping before your body has had a chance to tell you it was satisfied with the first.

To slow down the pace of eating, take 30 minutes for meals and 15 minutes for snacks.

Put down your utensil between bites. Savor each bite. Do not put it back into food until you have swallowed what is in your mouth.

Count your chews per bite. Take at least 15 chews per bite. When 3/4 of the meal is finished, stop eating for five minutes. At the end of this time, if you feel like eating more, continue. If you feel satisfied, stop and congratulate yourself.

If you want to take a second helping, wait 10 minutes before serving yourself seconds.

2. Eat in one location and set a full place setting for any food or beverage you take. This reduces the number of places you associate with food and makes it difficult to "eat on the run." Make eating a special occurrence, and take time to enjoy it. You deserve it.

Do not participate in other activities while eating. No television, radio, telephone, or reading while eating. Without these distractions, you will feel like you are getting more out of each mouthful.

Use a luncheon plate or dessert plate for your meal rather than a full-size dinner plate. It will seem like you are getting more food than you really are.

Know your portion sizes. Use a scale and measuring cups as you begin and until you feel comfortable "eyeballing" your correct portion.

Do not serve food family style. Instead serve your plate from the pots and pans in which it was cooked. You will be better able to resist taking seconds, and if you decide on seconds, you have to get up to refill your plate.

If you are tempted to nibble after you have finished your meal, have someone else in the family clear the plates and put away leftovers.

3. Store food out of sight and out of reach.
Food-proof your house.
Do not leave any food on the counter or table in plain view—this tests willpower too much. Put it away and use containers you can't see through.

Store food, especially problem foods, in an inconvenient place.

Spend less time in places or situations where you are surrounded by food.

Avoid purchasing food that you tend to overeat, especially

high calorie foods. You will be less likely to snack if it requires a walk to the grocery store rather than a walk to the kitchen.

4. Change purchasing and preparation habits.
Cut down the amount of food available to you at meals by preparing smaller portions. Prepare only one serving per person.

Avoid buying food that you tend to overeat. Write out a shopping list before you go to the supermarket. Buy only the items on the list.

Avoid shopping for groceries when you are hungry. If your stomach is growling, you will be more likely to buy high calorie foods and snacks.

If you nibble while preparing a meal, make the next meal when you're not hungry. Then, re-heat at the usual meal time. This will reduce the temptation to nibble.

5. Make specific plans to change eating habits.
Keep a written food diary of eating patterns. Does any pattern of overeating emerge that you could change? Set aside time each day to think ahead and plan your food intake for the next day. Develop the habit of eating three or more balanced meals daily. Never skip a meal. (This could be dangerous if you take diabetic pills or insulin.) Most people find if they skip one meal, they just overeat at the next one.

Leave a little bit of food on your plate. Many people feel compelled to finish everything on their plate because of childhood "clean plate" training. This technique is especially helpful when eating in restaurants.

Drink a glass of water, tomato or vegetable juice or a cup of broth before meals to help curb your appetite.

Keep a supply of low calorie foods on hand—diet gelatin, raw vegetables, or diet pop.

Reward yourself with non-food goodies for accomplishing a new behavior.

Record your weight once a week. Avoid weighing yourself

too often. It is easy to become discouraged if you don't see results on the scale each day.

6. **Set goals to gradually increase your energy expenditure.** Keep written records of your exercise.

7. **Avoid fad diets.** New and supposedly miraculous ways of losing weight are publicized almost every day. They are popular because they promise weight loss quickly and without effort. Some of the characteristics of fad diets are:

Temporary—a new fad diet seems to appear every week.

Irrational—most fad diets distort or ignore principles of good nutrition and defy the laws of nature. They may overemphasize one food or food group, assigning almost magical powers to it. They can be medically dangerous.

Something for nothing—beware of the "calories don't count" types of diet.

Limited variety—they often provide few food choices and are difficult to stick to for any length of time.

Off target—fad diets often cause loss of muscle and body water instead of fat. The water is quickly replaced when the diet is over. The muscle lost causes loss of body tone.

Expensive!—there is usually some "special" product or food or book necessary for the "success" of the diet.

YOU CAN DO IT!

For weight loss to be successful and permanent, do the following:

- Eat 250 to 500 calories per day less than usual in a balanced meal plan. Spread your calories over the whole day. Don't eat all your calories at one meal.

- Participate in regular exercise to burn additional calories and increase mental and physical well-being.

- Identify problem eating behaviors and make gradual changes.

- Maintain a gradual weight loss of 1/2 to 1 to 2 pounds per week until you reach your weight goal.

- When you reach your goal weight, keep healthy eating habits and regular exercise a permanent part of your lifestyle. Enjoy the new you!

CHAPTER 7

EXERCISE FOR THE HEALTH OF IT

Gene, like so many of us, always meant to start an exercise program, but he always had an excuse: "not enough time . . . too cold . . . too hot . . . too tired." Now that he has diabetes, Gene thinks differently about exercise. Diabetes and exercise are high on his priority list, and now he easily fits in a 30 minute walk 3 to 4 times a week.

In the beginning, Gene's motives for exercising were to lose weight and lower his blood glucose. But Gene also noticed that he felt better because he was taking care of himself. His self-image improved. He soon realized he had more energy and felt more relaxed than he had in years.

WHY IS EXERCISE IMPORTANT FOR SOMEONE WITH DIABETES?

• Exercise can lower blood glucose levels and improve your body's ability to use glucose.

Working muscles use glucose more effectively than resting muscles. Studies show that regular exercise increases the number of insulin receptor sites on cells. This increases the body's sensitivity to insulin. Because of this, if you take a diabetes pill or insulin you may be able to lower your dosage.

Physical fitness can also help reverse the resistance to insulin that occurs with obesity.

• Exercise can help reduce risk factors that can lead to heart disease, a major threat to people with Type II diabetes. Exercise helps lower fats (cholesterol and triglycerides) in the blood. It is also the best way to increase the amount of high density lipoprotein (HDL) cholesterol, the type of cholesterol that protects against heart disease.

• Exercise helps lower blood pressure. High blood pressure (hypertension) contributes to many problems that occur with diabetes, such as kidney and eye damage.

• Exercise burns up calories. Especially when you eat fewer calories, exercise can help you lose weight. By eating 500 calories per day less, you can lose a pound of fat per week. Now by adding exercises that burn up 250 calories per day you can lose another 1/2 pound per week. That's a total of 1 1/2 pounds of fat a week!

• Exercising when losing weight helps to keep and build muscle, which burns more calories than fat. Regular exercise makes weight maintenance easier.

ARE YOU READY?

Before you begin an exercise plan, answer the following questions. They will help you know if it's necessary to check with your doctor before you set up your personal program.

Do you have high blood pressure?	YES	NO
Have you ever had a heart attack?	YES	NO
Have you had episodes of severe dizziness, fainting, or blackouts?	YES	NO
Do you ever experience chest pain (angina), pain in the jaw, neck, or arm, or extreme shortness of breath?	YES	NO
Do you have back or joint pain, such as from arthritis or other diseases?	YES	NO
Do you ever have shakiness, dizziness, sweating, blurry vision or headaches? (These are signs of hypoglycemia or low blood glucose.)	YES	NO
Do you smoke?	YES	NO
Do you have numbness, tingling, burning, or pain in your feet?	YES	NO
Do you have pain or cramping in your calf muscles when you walk short distances?	YES	NO
Have you been told that you have changes in your eyes or kidneys caused by diabetes?	YES	NO
Has your blood glucose been higher than your target range for the last few months?	YES	NO

THE FIRST STEP

If you answered **yes** to any of the above questions, you may have a medical problem that needs to be looked into before you begin exercising. In some individuals who have higher risks for heart disease, a stress electrocardiogram may need to be done to determine whether it is advisable to exercise.

STEP TWO—OUTLINE A PLAN

How regularly have you been exercising?

Seldom?
(less than
once a week)

Fairly often?
(once or twice
a week)

Often?
(three to five
times a week)

If you are not physically active, you must proceed with a carefully paced program. Even if you've been fairly active, don't expect yourself to do too much too quickly.

Choose an activity or activities that you enjoy.

Below are just a few suggestions. Check those that appeal to you. If you normally like to exercise outdoors, think about what you might do indoors when weather does not permit safe exercise outdoors. Or simply for variety, consider a few different activities for different seasons of the year.

_____ Walking

_____ Water Aerobics

_____ Jumping Rope

_____ Mini-trampoline

_____ Cross Country Skiing

_____ Bicycling, outdoor or stationary

_____ Aerobics Classes (including low-impact aerobics)

_____ Ice Skating

_____ Treadmill

_____ Rowing Machine

_____ Swimming

_____ Jogging

_____ Roller Skating

_____ Dancing

Wear clothing that is comfortable and suited to the type of exercise you will be doing. Clothing that stretches and is loose-fitting will be more comfortable.

You need to be especially careful to protect your feet. Be sure you have the right shoes. They should be appropriate for the activities you choose. But more important, they should be right for your feet.

Schedule your exercise at a time of day that is realistic for you, when you re most likely to do it.

. . . Shade in the times of day that you are locked into activities such as work, meetings, etc. Can you walk during lunch break? Exercise while other family members make dinner? If you work at night, can you exercise before or after work?

Use this chart to identify times for exercise.

Time	M	T	W	TH	F	S	S
A.M. 12-1							
1-2							
2-3							
3-4							
4-5							
5-6							
6-7							
7-8							
8-9							
9-10							
10-11							
11-12							
P.M. Noon-1							
1-2							
2-3							
3-4							
4-5							
5-6							
6-7							
7-8							
8-9							
9-10							
10-11							
11-12							

WHAT IS AN EXERCISE PROGRAM?

When you plan your exercise, think about three parts: the warm-up, the training portion (activity of your choice from page 65) and the cool-down. Each is important.

Warm-ups are done to prepare your body for the aerobics portion of the workout. Generally, a warm-up should last about 10 minutes. It includes stretching and flexibility exercises. Done properly, a warm-up can help prevent injury and reduce muscle soreness.

Two "don'ts" during warm-ups:

1. Don't bounce when you stretch. You will be more likely to strain a muscle.

2. Don't stretch to the point of pain. At that point you may have already injured a muscle. Stretch slowly and hold for 10 to 20 seconds at the point where you begin to feel the muscle pulling.

The training portion is the main event of your exercise program. The purpose is to strengthen your heart and lungs. It should include an activity that you can do nonstop for a set period of time and at a controlled, comfortable pace. Racquet ball, tennis, golf, etc., although enjoyable, are examples of start/stop activities. They will not be as helpful as continuous exercise in losing weight, improving endurance and controlling blood glucose.

If you have not been a regular exerciser, it is important that you begin slowly and gradually work up to harder work-outs. You will avoid needless pain, muscle soreness and injury. Even if you feel you could easily walk for an hour, build up to it.

Follow these guidelines during your training period:

Intensity: This refers to how hard you work during exercise. The best way to know how hard you are working is to check your pulse every 5 to 10 minutes during exercise, especially when you are just beginning an exercise program.

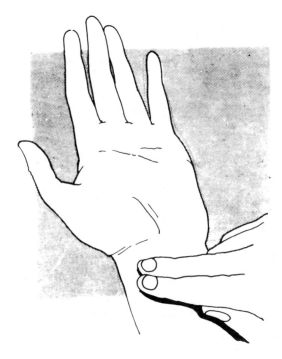

PULSE TAKING

Here's an easy way to take your pulse. You'll need a watch or clock with a second hand.

1. As shown in the illustration above, rest the pointer and middle fingers on the bone at your wrist.

2. Drop those fingers about 1/4 inch down the wrist. You should be able to find your pulse there.

3. With your fingers resting gently over the pulse, count the number of beats you feel for 10 seconds. Use this number as a guide for your target heart rate.

To get the maximum heart and lung benefit from your exercise program, your heart must reach and maintain a certain number of beats per minute. This is called your target heart rate. Take your pulse during and immediately after you stop exercising. Count only for 10 seconds, because your heart rate will slow down drastically after just 15 seconds.

TARGET
HEART RATE CHART

AGE	BEATS/10 SEC.	BEATS/MINUTE
30	19 - 24	114 - 143
35	19 - 23	111 - 139
40	18 - 23	108 - 135
45	18 - 22	105 - 131
50	17 - 21	102 - 128
55	17 - 21	99 - 124
60	16 - 20	96 - 120
65	16 - 19	93 - 116
70	15 - 19	90 - 113
75	15 - 18	87 - 109
80	14 - 18	84 - 105
85	14 - 17	81 - 101

My target heart rate is _____ beats per 10 seconds.

If your pulse while exercising is below the recommended level, pick up your pace slightly. If your pulse is too high, slow your pace, but do not stop. Stopping would slow your heart to a "resting" rate and you would lose the training effect.

If checking your pulse is too difficult, just listen to your body to determine how hard you are working. If you are gasping for air and breathing rapidly, you are working too hard. You need to slow your pace until you are breathing deeply, but no longer huffing and puffing. You should be able to carry on a conversation during the activity. (Good luck swimmers!)

Some blood pressure medications (beta-blockers, in particular) control the heart rate. If you are taking this type of medicine, you will need to use the exertion scale.

Exercise Intensity	
Perceived Exertion	**Comment**
Very, very light	This intensity is of little value.
Very light	
Light but noticeable	GO! This intensity is just right.
Moderate	
Somewhat hard	
Hard	STOP! This intensity is much too hard.
Very hard breathing heavily.	

Duration: This is the length of time you exercise in one session. This will be decided by your current level of fitness and your goals for exercising. Is your goal to feel better? Have more energy? To lose weight? To lower blood glucose? To run a marathon?

If you are just beginning, the duration may only be 3 to 5 minutes at first. In order to achieve heart and lung fitness and overall conditioning, gradually increase your time by 3 to 5 minutes a week until you can exercise non-stop for 20 to 30 minutes. Longer periods are even more beneficial for weight loss or competition, such as a race.

Frequency: This is the number of times you exercise per week. The minimum should be 3 times per week. If weight loss is your goal, you may choose to exercise five or six times a week. You may also want to vary activities so you use different muscle groups each day, for example, swimming one day and biking the next.

If you are just beginning a program, consider exercise sessions every other day to allow time for your muscles to recover. As you become more fit, you will be able to increase the frequency without pain or strain.

If you increase the duration or intensity of your exercise and find it too strenuous continue at that level an extra week and then go on to the next pattern. You do not have to be doing 30 minutes of exercise within a set time period. Increase at a pace that is comfortable and safe for you!

Remember to do stretching exercises before the walking warm-up and after the walking cool-down.

Cool down: The final activity is the cool down period. This allows your body to gradually slow down after the training period. Slow walking and stretching exercises are good ways to cool down. The cool down period should last about 10 to 12 minutes, or longer if you like.

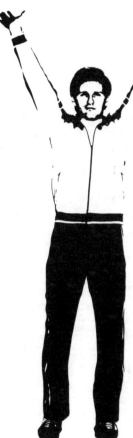

Examples of Stretching Exercises

Overhead Stretch
- Stand, feet shoulder width apart, arms at sides.
- Raise arms out to sides until fully extended overhead. Hold stretch, return arms to sides. Inhale while raising arms, exhale while lowering arms.

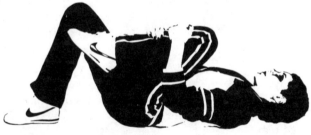

Knees To Chest
- Lie on back knees bent, feet flat on the floor.
- Pull right knee to chest and hold with both hands. Lower foot back to floor. Aternate knees. Keep lower back on the floor throughout movement and keep chin tucked in.

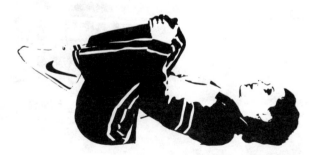

- Pull both knees to chest by holding knees in both hands. Spread knees apart, hold, lower feet back to floor.

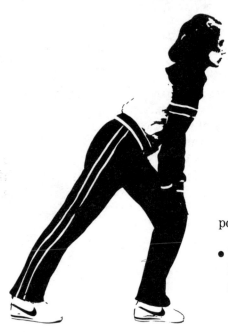

Calf Stretch
- Stand in forward stride position, toes pointed forward, as if standing in a straight line.
- Lean forward bending front knee, keeping back leg straight. Stretch gently until you feel the muscle in the calf of your back leg stretch, hold, release.

Knee Extension
- Lie on your back, with your knees bent and together.
- Rest arms at sides, chin tucked into chest.
- Bring one knee into chest, extend leg, lower back down to floor, return to starting position.
- Switch legs.

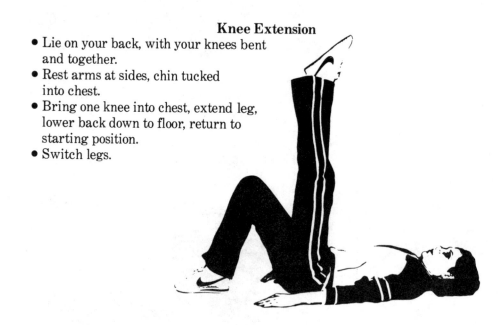

Exercise illustrations and instructions reproduced through the courtesy of SHAPE, Inc., a program of Park Nicollet Medical Foundation.

YOUR EXERCISE RECORD

Example

	S	M	T	W	TH	F	S
Week 1	Walk 5 min.		Walk 5 min.		Bike 5 min.		Walk 5 min.
Week 2	Walk 7 min.		Walk 7 min.		Walk 10 min.		Bike 10 min.

My Record

	S	M	T	W	TH	F	S
Week 1							
Week 2							
Week 3							
Week 4							
Week 5							
Week 6							

(Goal: 20-30 minutes of continuous activity.)

To monitor the glucose lowering effects of exercise, we recommend testing your blood glucose before and after exercise. People respond differently to exercise. Some may see an immediate drop after and some see a drop hours later. Some may not see a change at all directly related to exercise. However, those people often have improved blood glucose levels as they lose weight or make other lifestyle changes.

WHAT ABOUT RISKS ASSOCIATED WITH EXERCISING?

While you hear much about the physical and psychological benefits of exercise, you don't usually hear about the risks, especially if you have a chronic disease, such as arthritis, high blood pressure, or diabetes, or physical disabilities.

Your doctor may be able to suggest safe activities for you or refer you to an exercise specialist who can tailor a program for your specific needs.

Risks most associated with exercise and diabetes are:

1. **Foot injury:** While walking is generally a safe exercise for most people, if you have any foot deformities, nerve damage, or circulatory changes, walking may cause further damage. Always look at your feet after exercise, paying attention to any areas that are red, hot, blistering, swollen, or tender. Seek medical advise immediately if such problems persist. Wearing proper shoes can help prevent foot injuries.

2. **Muscle injury:** This can occur with almost any type of exercise. It is important to rest the injured area. Consult your doctor if you are concerned that you have a more serious type of injury. Warm-up and cool-down stretching exercises will help prevent muscle injury.

3. **Hypoglycemia:** Since exercise improves the glucose lowering effects of diabetes medicines (pills and insulin), you may need to monitor blood glucoses before and after exercise, especially if you exercise during the peak action time of the medication. Carry quick-acting, carbohydrate—containing food with you and use it if you begin having

symptoms such as shakiness, sweating, blurred vision, dizziness, or headaches. These are symptoms of hypoglycemia, which can occur during exercise. (See page 96 for more information about hypoglycemia.)

4. **Dehydration:** Especially on those hot, summer days, drink plenty of fluids to replace what you lose during exercise.

5. **Silent heart attacks:** People with diabetes who have impaired nerve sensations sometimes don't have typical signs of heart attacks such as chest pain. If these people over-exercise, they can be at risk for a heart attack they don't feel.

6. **Worsening of already present diabetes complications:** This is particularly related to eye and nerve damage. If you have been told you have any of these, strenuous jarring exercises need to be avoided. Nerve damage could block the body's ability to feel pain from overdoing it or from injury. You will need a specially designed program to prevent further damage.

CAUTION SIGNS

Seek medical help immediately if any of the following occurs:

1. Unusual heart action. For example, irregular beats, fluttering, or sudden slow pulse.

2. Pain or pressure in the chest, arm, or jaw.

3. Dizziness or lightheadedness. (This could be a symptom of low blood glucose but also can be a symptom of heart or circulation problems.)

4. Cold sweat.

5. Extreme breathlessness or shortness of breath.

6. Rapid heart beat five to ten minutes after exercise has stopped.

7. Steady joint pain lasting more than two hours.

8. Prolonged fatigue, undue stiffness, or pain in the joints even 24 hours later.

SUMMING UP

We know beginning an exercise program can be difficult, especially if you've never exercised before. But is it a very important part of treating your diabetes—just as diet, weight loss and medication are important. We want you to take it seriously and do it cautiously. Exercise with the approval of your doctor. Monitor your progress. Seek out an exercise class if you need the structure, support of others, set times, and accountability. It all can help ensure progress and success.

CHAPTER 8

BLOOD GLUCOSE MONITORING: YOUR MIRROR OF CONTROL

Monitoring is a marvelous tool for actually "seeing" what is happening with blood glucose values.

Testing your blood for glucose yourself is an easy, convenient way to get immediate feedback on your diabetes management. It involves pricking your finger to obtain a drop of blood and placing the drop on a chemically treated pad. (To many people, this procedure sounds painful, but technology is becoming so advanced that it hardly hurts at all.) The color change of the pad will tell you, within a range, what your blood glucose level is at that moment. There are also meters that will "read" the test pad and give you the exact level of blood glucose.

Monitoring means keeping track of your test results. Although some folks like to use their home computers to store information, a simple record book will do just fine!

Blood monitoring is valuable in managing Type II diabetes. You and your health care team will use the results to assess your overall diabetes control, decide on the best form of treatment and make medication or diet adjustments. It will be the basis for your day-to-day decisions. Good decision-making includes knowing when to contact your doctor about blood glucose levels, choosing healthy foods, and knowing when and how long to exercise, as well as managing stress.

In a sense, you need to do externally what your body can no longer do internally. Before you had diabetes, your body could automatically monitor the blood glucose and adjust the amount of insulin and glucose released to keep the levels between 60 and 160 mg/dl. Now you have to make adjustments in what you do to control blood glucose. The only way to know if what you are doing is working is to test your blood yourself and record the results.

When you record each blood test result you will soon begin to see that your blood glucose levels may follow certain patterns. This information can help you plan your meals, exercise, and medication in an effort to keep blood glucose levels as near normal as possible.

If you're just getting started, here's what you need to perform a test. Your blood testing equipment consists of:

- Test strips
- Finger pricking device
- Lancets
- Record book
- Meter (optional)

The next step is to be trained by a health professional who is experienced with blood glucose monitoring. Blood testing can be expensive and accuracy of information is crucial so it makes sense that you are trained to do it correctly, right from the start.

WHAT YOU NEED TO KNOW ABOUT BLOOD TESTING PRODUCTS

Test strips—There are several brands to choose from, so spend some time with a trained professional learning which kind is best for you.

The strips are used by comparing the test strip to a color chart after blood has been adequately applied and properly removed from a chemically treated pad.

Timing is crucial for an accurate test and varies by brand. Know the manufacturer's recommendations for the one you choose.

Meters—These are small, battery operated instruments that "read" the test strips and show a precise blood glucose value.

You may need a meter if you:

- are color blind
- have verified with a trained health professional or against laboratory values that you are interpreting the strips incorrectly.
- are using insulin and find your blood glucose levels vary significantly throughout the day.

Many people can do well without meters. If you're not sure, consider what you would do differently for your diabetes if you had an exact value rather than an approximate value. If you visually can tell the difference between the colors in the normal range and when it goes beyond, that may be all you need to know to tell if you are on the right track.

3. Devices that hold very sharp needles or lancets allow you to get a drop of blood with little or no pain. There are several on the market. They vary in ease of loading, depth of puncture, size, cost, and comfort. If you have the opportunity, try different devices before you buy one.

Note: Many insurance companies offer coverage for all or a portion of diabetes supplies. Submit your receipts or a copy of your bill to your insurance company for possible reimbursement.

SOME TIPS FOR TESTING YOUR BLOOD

1. Choose a site. Sides of the fingertips are recommended for people with Type II diabetes. Rotate sites to avoid tender, bruised fingers. (Toes are not recommended because of possible poor circulation or loss of sensitivity in your feet.)

2. Prepare the site by washing your hands with soap and warm water. Washing thoroughly helps prevent infection and will remove any sugar from food that could cause the reading to be falsely high. Warm water will increase blood flow to the area. Dry the area thoroughly. It is best not to use alcohol to clean the skin. If the alcohol is not completely dry, it can change the blood glucose reading as well as cause discomfort. It also dries the skin.

3. Puncture the site. When a large drop accumulates, allow it to hang from the puncture site. Then carefully place it on the test pad. With some products the blood must be dropped onto the pad, and with others it can be smeared. *If you have trouble getting enough blood, gently massage your hand and milk the finger. (You can try this before puncturing the skin as well as after.) Another option is to let your arm* *hang at your side for 30 seconds or more to allow blood to pool in the fingers.*

4. Cover the pad completely and uniformly. This is crucial for getting an accurate result. Timing and proper removal of the blood (if necessary for your method) also are important for accuracy.

It's a good idea to compare a test against a laboratory glucose test periodically so you know your technique is accurate. Take your supplies along to your doctor's appointment and do a test at the same time a lab test is drawn.

Your result may vary slightly from the lab. Blood drawn from a vein and spun down shows plasma glucose. When you test your blood, it is whole blood drawn from a capillary. Your results should be within 10 to 15 percent of the laboratory test.

5. Write down your results in a record book. That is the only way you can monitor changes over time.

HOW OFTEN DO YOU NEED TO TEST?

Remember that blood testing is a means of gathering information. It's not necessarily a reflection of whether you've done something "wrong" or you've been bad or good. You may want more information than someone else so you may choose to test frequently. You may need to test less often if your diabetes is stable and well controlled. For someone with Type II diabetes, it's important that you test often enough to collect the information you need to truly manage your diabetes well.

We recommend the following:

> . . .**Test a minimum of 2 days per week.** (Test on a weekday and weekend if your routine changes.)
>
> . . .**Test 2 to 3 times per day on the days you test—** before eating breakfast, before lunch and/or before supper and occasionally two hours after you begin a meal. (Blood glucose levels are at their highest one to two hours after a meal.)

Be your own investigator. Especially in the beginning, you will want to understand how your blood glucose is affected by different types and amounts of food, exercise, stress, illness, or changes in routine.

Test when you don't feel quite up to par and want to know if your blood glucose is related to that feeling. Always test when you are ill. Blood glucose is usually higher during illness or infection. If illness is prolonged, insulin may be necessary so healing can take place.

Makes notes in your record book if you think you can explain blood glucose levels at a given time. For example:

Date	Meds Time	A.M. BG	Morning Comments	Noon BG	Afternoon Comments	P.M. BG	Evening Comments
Sun.	8:00	100	Went out for breakfast	180	Walked 2 miles	120	2 hr. after meal b.g. 150
Mon.	7:30	80		—	Stressful meeting	210	ate dessert 2 hr. b.g. > 240 oh no!
Tues.	7:30	180	Sore throat, fever	320	Neg. ketones Saw doctor	320	Went to bed early
Sat.	8:30	150	Feeling better	—	Walked 2 miles	100	
Sun.	8:00	80	Skipped breakfast	11:00 40	Felt shaky and sweaty. Drank o.j.	100	

WHAT DO THE NUMBERS MEAN?

You will find blood testing more helpful if you know what your test result is in comparison with a normal or target range. And understanding the factors that may have influenced your test result will help you take action.

People without diabetes have enough insulin available so glucose can be taken in by the cells and used for energy. This means their blood glucose levels will always stay within normal ranges.

A normal range is defined as:

Fasting and before meals: 60 to 110 mg/dl

One to two hours after meals: at or below 160 mg/dl.

It makes no difference which type of diabetes a person has—the goal is to return blood glucose levels to normal or as near normal as possible to keep a person feeling well and at lower risk for diabetes complications. For example, if you cannot recognize symptoms of hypoglycemia, or if you have heart disease, it would be dangerous to have your blood glucose levels in the lower range of normal. For reasons like these, your doctor may modify your target blood glucose range to something like 80-140 mg/dl before meals and up to 180 mg/dl after meals.

Discuss a target range for your blood glucose with your doctor. Write it here. It will help you when you assess your control.

My target blood glucose range

Fasting and before meals _____ mg/dl.

1-2 hours after meals _____ mg/dl.

WHAT AFFECTS
THE RESULTS?

Some of the factors that may raise blood glucose levels are:

- Emotional stress, both good and bad
- Physical stress—injury, illness, surgery, pain, infection
- Food—type, amount, timing of meals or snacks
- Lack of activity or sedentary lifestyle
- Some medications, such as cortisone.

Some factors that may lower blood glucose levels are:

- Weight loss
- Limiting or avoiding foods with simple carbohydrates (desserts, etc.)
- Carefully following a meal plan
- Exercise/increased activity
- Some medications, particularly insulin and oral diabetes pills
- Relaxation

DO I NEED TO BE CONCERNED
IF THE NUMBERS ARE HIGH?

The answer is yes and maybe.

There is cause for great concern the longer glucose levels remain high. If diabetes is poorly controlled over many months to years, irrepairable damage to blood vessels and nerves can occur. That's why we urge you to take diabetes seriously and take action now. Treatment for high blood glucose (hyperglycemia) is what this book is primarily about.

If the blood levels are high and there is not enough insulin or it is not effective in moving glucose into the cells, ketones may be formed. These are acids formed when the body switches over to burning fat for energy. Because there is a problem with insulin, even this back-up energy source (fat) is ineffective. Ketones build up and can appear in the urine. A positive ketone test is like a flashing red light telling you your diabetes is getting out of control. You may need to change how you treat your diabetes.

This occurs more rapidly in people with Type I diabetes. Even though you are not as prone to this, you should know how and when to check your urine for ketones. It is a simple test done by dipping a chemically treated strip in the urine stream or a cup of urine, waiting an allotted amount of time, and comparing it with a color chart.

Test for ketones if:

1. Your blood glucose remains above 300 for several tests
2. You are ill
3. You have a sudden drop in weight.

Talk with your doctor or health care provider about what you should do if your blood glucose levels are high and your ketone test is positive.

When blood glucose levels occasionally are high (more than 160 mg/dl) and you can explain them, such as eating too much or at the wrong times, just getting back on your meal plan and regular schedule may correct the problem. Exercise will help too. A high glucose, even if it is occasional, should not be ignored and will become a concern if it happens repeatedly.

WHAT ABOUT LOW GLUCOSE LEVELS?

Should you be concerned about low blood glucose levels?

The answer is yes and no.

No, you do not need to be concerned if you are on diet only. It is extremely rare that your blood glucose will go too low.

Yes, if you take diabetes pills or insulin injections there is the risk of having low blood glucoses.

When blood glucose falls to below 60 mg/dl, you may have symptoms such as sweating, shaking, paleness, blurring vision, hunger, headache, dizziness or a racing heart. This is the way your body signals that it needs more glucose. If untreated, symptoms progress to impaired judgment and coordination and possibly loss of consciousness.

If you think your glucose may be low, test your blood to find out exactly what is going on.

See page 96 for treatment of hypoglycemia.

YOUR RECORD: WHAT DO YOU "SEE" IN THE MIRROR?

As you review your blood glucose records look for patterns. Analyze them and decide what you can do differently. Consider the following questions:

1. Are there trends from week to week?

2. Are the results higher, lower or within your recommended target range?

3. What factors may have influenced the results? Can you explain a high or a low blood glucose? Is this a pattern— such as consistently overeating at one time of the day?

4. How do blood glucose readings compare with others taken at the same time of the day?

5. How does your blood glucose change during the day?

6. What time of day does it tend to be the highest?

7. Is there a difference between weekdays and weekends?

8. Have you had any hypoglycemic (low blood glucose) reactions? What triggered them? Symptoms? Treatment? What was the blood glucose level?

Then consider the following:

1. What do you think you could do to improve your blood glucose? If you can see a pattern of high glucose levels that you can explain, then you can choose to change your behavior.

2. How much has your weight changed? Is there a correlation with blood glucose levels? As weight comes down, we hope to see your blood glucose come down, too.

3. How carefully are you following your meal plan? Does it make a difference in your blood glucose results? Is there room for improvement? Keep track of your blood glucose results on days you "blew it" also. This could be a motivator in itself to help you stay on your plan.

4. Are you exercising? Test your blood glucoses before and again an hour after exercise so you can see if exercise helps lower it.

5. If blood glucose levels are high at the same time of the day, such as before your evening meal, can you fit your exercise in during the afternoon? Or could you change the timing or amount of your lunch or afternoon snack? (People taking insulin should consult with health care professionals before cutting out food or altering their schedule.)

CONTACT OR SEE YOUR DOCTOR IF:

• Hypoglycemic reactions (low blood glucose, insulin reaction) occur. If you have frequent or severe reactions, you may need a decrease in your medication dose or to rearrange your meal plan.

• Blood glucose tests remain unchanged or get worse after 10 to 15 pounds of weight loss, following your diet and exercise program, or after a change in medication dose. It helps to clarify with your health care team how much time should elapse before contacting them if there is no improvement. *With diet, exercise, and weight loss it may be appropriate to wait three to six months, especially if glucose test results show a downward trend. If you're taking diabetes pills or insulin, your doctor may want to hear from you after one to four weeks.*

•You are not feeling well and think it is related to your diabetes such as symptoms of hyperglycemia or long-term complications, including numbness, tingling in the feet, etc. Be sure to tell your doctor what your blood glucose levels are, as well as your symptoms.

• You are concerned about your blood glucose readings.

CHAPTER 9

DIABETES PILLS: A JUMP START FOR NATURE'S INSULIN

In 1955, scientists discovered a group of drugs that improve the body's ability to use insulin. These pills are called oral hypoglycemic agents or sometimes just oral agents. They are not oral insulin and shouldn't be thought of as a substitute for insulin.

Your body's own insulin must be available for diabetes pills to work. Pills don't help people with Type I diabetes, since there is no natural insulin present.

WHY TAKE DIABETES PILLS?

Weight loss, healthy eating and exercise are the first steps to lowering blood glucose. These are also positive changes to make in your life. For lots of people, this program works, but sometimes it doesn't.

Mary is one example. She was doing fine with exercise and changes in her lifestyle. She lost some weight and her blood glucose improved, but still wasn't in the target range she and her diabetes team had set. What should she do now? Her doctor prescribed diabetes pills and her blood glucose levels went down again.

WHEN ARE THEY USED?

Diabetes pills are prescribed when blood glucose is no longer adequately controlled by the present treatment plan of diet and exercise. The usual pattern is to start with a low dose of a pill and to adjust as needed to for control.

Your doctor will work with you to find the one that best suits your needs and effectively lowers your blood glucose. When a person with Type II diabetes first uses oral agents, the pills seem to stimulate the pancreas to release more insulin. In the long run, however, the pills don't seem to cause an increase in insulin levels. Recent studies have shown oral agents help lower blood glucose by increasing the effectiveness of insulin when it reaches the cells.

Experts sometimes disagree about who benefits from oral agents. Most agree, however, that oral agents should NOT be used in Type I diabetes or by a pregnant or breast-feeding woman or by those who are allergic to sulfa compounds. They also should not be used if a person has liver or kidney disease, because the body would not be able to dispose of the drug. It would accumulate and severe hypoglycemia could result.

Doctors also agree that nutrition and weight control are the primary methods for controlling Type II diabetes and oral agents should be used only when dietary management has been unsuccessful. If the oral agents do not result in good blood glucose control after a trial period of about 3 to 6 months, they should be stopped.

Commonly accepted guidelines for the use of oral agents are as follows:

• Only people with Type II diabetes should be given oral agents.

• Oral agents are tried after meal planning, weight loss and regular exercise have not been successful in providing reasonable blood glucose control.

• Use of oral agents is continued if blood glucose levels are reasonably controlled (usually under 120 mg fasting and under 180 mg one to two hours after eating). If high blood glucose persists despite a maximum dose of an oral agent, the person with Type II diabetes should start on insulin.

SIDE EFFECTS OF ORAL AGENTS

As with any medication, you might have some side effects from oral agents. Fortunately, these problems don't happen very often, but you should be aware of what could happen.

Probably the most common side effect is low blood glucose—hypoglycemia. Since the job of oral agents is to lower your blood glucose, it could go too low if you skip or delay meals or if you are on too large a dose. This isn't usually a serious problem, and it's more likely to occur if you take insulin shots. If your blood glucose goes too low, you can eat a small amount of food to bring it back up. (See hypoglycemia treatment, page 97.)

Other side effects of diabetes pills could include an allergic reaction, causing a rash, hives, or upset stomach. You might also have bloating, cramping, and a loss of appetite. If you have any of these symptoms, tell your doctor.

In the rare individual, the combination of alcohol and oral agents can cause a syndrome of headache, facial flushing, and nausea. If this happens to you, you will not be able to drink alcohol while taking this drug. A different oral agent may not cause that reaction.

You may have heard that diabetes pills can increase your risk of heart disease. This is not true. One study carried out in the 1960s reported a higher risk of heart disease, but studies since then have not found a connection between diabetes pills and heart disease. The American Diabetes Association investigated this question carefully and has determined oral agents are safe.

ARE THERE DIFFERENT KINDS OF ORAL AGENTS?

All oral agents currently available in the U.S. are related to sulfa drugs, which are commonly used to fight infections. The scientific name for oral agents is "sulfonylurea agents." Four oral agents have been available in the United States for some time: Orinase®, Dymelor®, Tolinase®, and Diabinese®. Two other oral agents that are 100 to 200 times as potent as those mentioned above have recently been marketed in the United States: Glucotrol® and DiaBeta®/Micronase®. (They are the same drug but different brand names.) Their superior strength makes it possible to give them in smaller doses.

The different kinds of oral agents are taken in different daily doses. They also act for different periods of time. Work closely with your doctor to find the dose that works best for you.

It's very important that you use medications exactly as your doctor tells you. Even though you feel perfectly fine, you still need the medication—just as you would need a blood pressure pill or an antibiotic. On the other hand, if you have any problems because of the medication, be sure to tell your doctor about it immediately.

ORAL MEDICATIONS

Trade Name	Generic Name	Duration of Activity	Usual Daily Dose	Schedule for Taking
Orinase®	Tolbutamide	6-12	500-3000 mg.	2 — 3 times daily
Diabinese®	Chlorpropamide	24-72	100-500 mg.	once daily
Dymelor®	Acetohexamide	12-16	250-1500 mg.	1 — 2 times daily
Tolinase®	Tolazamide	12-18	100-1000 mg.	1 — 2 times daily
DiaBeta®	Glyburide	24	1.25-20 mg.	1 — 2 times daily
Micronase®	Glyburide	24	1.25-20 mg.	1 — 2 times daily
Glucotrol®	Glipizide	24	2.5-40 mg.	1 — 2 times daily

CHAPTER 10

INSULIN: GIVING YOUR BODY A BREAK

Sometimes meal planning, exercise, and even oral agents aren't enough to control blood glucose levels. In these instances, people with Type II diabetes need to take insulin.

It seems odd, doesn't it, that you need insulin? If the pancreas still makes insulin, why would adding more insulin help?

Think of it like this: Your pancreas makes less insulin than it used to, and you have fewer receptor sites on your cells for that insulin to attach to. Also, you may be resistant to the insulin your body makes. Adding more insulin increases the chances enough insulin will attach to the receptor sites to allow glucose into the cells.

The fact that you need insulin does not mean you did anything wrong or that your diabetes is worse. We can't emphasize this enough. Some people just need to take insulin to control blood glucose. You still need to follow your meal plan and exercise regularly.

WHAT WILL THIS MEAN FOR YOU?

It's only natural to feel a little afraid if you need to begin taking insulin. Some people are afraid the shots will hurt. Others wonder how they will fit insulin injections into their lives. Others feel guilty if they haven't been taking good care of their diabetes. They think this is why they have to take insulin.

We understand these feelings, but insulin injections can become as normal a part of your daily routine as brushing your teeth. We know this is difficult to believe, but insulin shots are seldom painful. The needles today are very short and thin.

At first, when you start taking insulin, you may need to make some adjustments. You might have to get up a few minutes earlier in the morning, or remember to eat your meals on time. But with help from your diabetes team and your family and friends, taking insulin will quickly become routine.

You will soon begin to see that insulin is another part of your healthy lifestyle. It doesn't mean you are sick; you take it to stay healthy.

WHAT IS INSULIN?

Insulin is a hormone produced in your pancreas. Its role is to help glucose get into your cells where it can be used for energy. Insulin is a molecule made up of 51 building blocks called amino acids.

We all know that insulin is made by our pancreas, but what about the insulin that is injected? Where does that come from?

Until just a few years ago we got all of our insulin from the pancreas of cows or pigs; insulin from these animals is almost identical to the insulin we produce in our bodies, differing by one amino acid for pork insulin and by three amino acids for beef insulin. These two kinds of insulins worked fine most of the time. However, with the increasing demand for insulin, it was projected that soon there would not be enough insulin produced from animal sources. That would mean some who needed it would not be able to get it.

Fortunately scientists discovered how to make insulin in the laboratory. We call this human insulin because its structure is exactly like the insulin produced in our bodies. One process researchers use to make insulin is really very interesting. It's called recombinant DNA technology.

Scientists have figured out which genes of the body are responsible for making insulin. Genes are small units of DNA protein that can be compared to blueprints. They are the guides for building our bodies. Scientists can copy these blueprints and insert this copy into bacteria. The chemical machinery of the bacteria cell will follow this blueprint for human insulin and actually manufacture insulin identical to that normally found in human beings.

Another way to make human insulin is to modify pork insulin by taking out the one amino acid that makes it different from human insulin and replacing it with the one that does.

It is reassuring to know that because of these technologies, there will be an adequate supply of insulin available.

HOW MUCH INSULIN WILL YOU HAVE TO TAKE?

Each individual needs an insulin dose designed especially for him or her. Your doctor will probably have you take a small dosage at first and see how that works. Some people with Type II diabetes may take just one shot a day, but most people take two shots of insulin a day to control their blood glucose.

Two shots a day offer more flexibility for your daily routine. Usually one shot is taken before breakfast and another before your evening meal. In most instances, each shot will be a combination of short-acting insulin (regular) and intermediate-acting insulin (NPH or Lente).

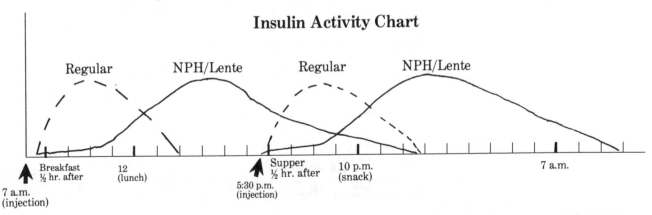

Insulin Activity Chart

	Begins	Peaks	Lasts
Short Acting (Regular)	15-30 min.	2-4 hrs.	5-7 hrs.
Intermediate Acting (NPH or Lente)	2-4 hrs.	6-12 hrs.	Up to 24 hrs.

Regular insulin, which is short acting, will help you use the food you are about to eat. NPH or Lente, the intermediate acting, will serve as a background insulin. Taking combined doses of insulin mimics to a degree the way a pancreas releases insulin: a little bit all day long and more after a meal.

HOW WILL YOU KNOW WHAT TO DO?

Insulin affects important aspects of your life—mainly when you eat and exercise. It is one medication you need to learn how to use. You cannot just follow instructions on a bottle of insulin, as you would when you swallow a pill. That's why when you start taking insulin you will need education about how to use it and when to take it. This will usually involve several sessions with a nurse educator and a dietitian.

You will learn:

1. How to prepare and take your insulin.

2. How insulin works.

3. How to check your blood glucose if you're not already doing it.

4. How to balance your food and insulin.

5. How to balance food and insulin with exercise.

These sessions are a good time to ask questions. If anything seems unclear to you, be sure to ask for a complete explanation.

HYPOGLYCEMIA OR "INSULIN REACTIONS"

As with oral agents, the purpose of insulin is to lower your glucose. Sometimes these glucose levels can go too low. This is called hypoglycemia or, if you are on insulin, an insulin reaction.

Several things can bring on an insulin reaction: too much

insulin, too much unplanned activity or exercise, or not enough food.

If your insulin dose is too high, it may need to be decreased. If you exercise a lot more than usual, you may need to eat extra food. If you are not eating enough food, you may need to adjust your meal plan or insulin. (If you're trying to lose weight, you probably don't need to eat more food. In that case, the insulin can be adjusted to match the amount of food you are eating.)

Insulin reactions can be serious. But if you know the symptoms of a reaction, you can do something before it gets dangerous. The symptoms of an insulin reaction include:

- Sweating
- Shakiness
- Dizziness
- Headaches
- Blurry vision
- Rapid heart beat
- Confusion
- Sleepiness

If you feel any of these symptoms and think it might be a reaction, test your blood first to make sure. If your blood glucose is below 80 eat a food containing simple sugar (carbohydrate). When you test and your blood glucose is 60 or less, treat it even though you may not have any symptoms. A food or beverage that contains simple sugar (carbohydrate) will work fastest.

The following are some suggestions:

- a small box of raisins
- 5-6 LifeSavers®
- 2 or 3 glucose tablets
- 4 or 5 small sugar cubes
- 1/2 cup fruit juice or regular soda pop
- 3 graham crackers
- 1 small piece of fruit

After treating a hypoglycemic reaction, wait 10 to 15 minutes. If you still have symptoms treat with the same amount again—about 60 calories. Then wait another 10 to 15 minutes. Test your blood. If symptoms are still present or your blood glucose remains under 60, contact your doctor.

There are premeasured gels and tablets on the market for treating hypoglycemia. They are convenient to carry in your pocket or purse or in the glove compartment of your car. Check with your pharmacist or diabetes products store about different brands. They also help prevent overtreating a hypoglycemic reaction.

It's tempting to want to eat an entire candy bar when you have a reaction. What a good excuse to eat sugar! But try to resist that temptation. A whole candy bar (or ice cream cone, or piece of pie) probably will make your blood glucose go sky high.

Always wear some form of identification stating you have diabetes. Be sure to tell your family and friends about insulin reactions and what they can do if they see you having signs of a reaction coming on. Sometimes, a person having an insulin reaction can appear drunk, and if the people you're with don't understand what's happening, they might not be able to help you.

IN SUMMARY

Insulin will help you manage your diabetes, and if your diabetes is in control, you'll feel better. It's like any of the other things you do by choice to live a healthier life: brushing and flossing your teeth or eating less salt, for example. Sometimes we resist these healthy habits because they take too much time or we can't remember to do them. But deep down, we know these things are good for us.

Living a healthy life with diabetes involves doing a few extra things we didn't do before. Taking insulin might be one of those things. If so, it's a positive force in your new, healthier life.

CHAPTER 11

AN OVERVIEW OF COMPLICATIONS

In the past, we thought people with Type II diabetes didn't have as many or as severe long-term health problems as individuals with Type I diabetes. Recent statistics tell us this is not—*definitely not*—true. Therefore, it's important for people with Type II diabetes to be informed about possible complications so they can avoid or reduce the risks.

WHAT ARE LONG-TERM COMPLICATIONS?

"Long-term" complications are those that can occur as a result of having diabetes for a period of time. In many instances, long-term refers to 5-10 years after diabetes develops. This is especially true for eye and kidney disease, but it is not always true for all diabetes complications. Some problems may be obvious when Type II diabetes is diagnosed—especially nerve damage.

The long-term complications of diabetes occur mainly because of damage to blood vessels. The body has literally hundreds of miles of blood vessels, some of them very small and other fairly large. Diabetes can damage any blood vessel in the body, but some seem to be at greater risk than others.

The problems caused by blood vessel damage are related to the size of the vessel and the area of the body in which the problem develops. Problems in the eyes, kidneys, and nerves are related to damage to the small blood vessels. Small blood vessel damage is called *microvascular* disease. Problems in the heart, feet, and brain are caused by damage to the large blood vessels, which is called *macrovascular* disease.

DOES DIABETES DAMAGE BLOOD VESSELS?

Abnormal blood glucose levels are thought to be the main factor in causing damage. The theory is that blood vessels bathed with abnormally high blood glucose for many months or years will become damaged.

Various research studies, some with animals and some with humans, have looked at the effect of blood glucose levels on the development of blood vessel damage. A famous study done in dogs with diabetes showed that dogs with high blood glucose levels had more damage to their eyes than dogs with normal blood glucose levels. A 20 year study of humans with diabetes done in Belgium showed that individuals with normal or near normal fasting blood glucose levels over the years ended up with the least eye, kidney and nerve problems related to diabetes, whereas individuals with high fasting blood glucose levels developed more diabetes-related problems.

It may be that other factors contribute to causing complications such as high blood fat levels and high blood pressure. Heredity may also play a part in determining who gets complications and who doesn't.

As yet we do not have all the answers. Research is continuing on the problems of diabetes. Many studies are being done to help us learn more about complications: why they happen and how we can prevent them from occurring.

In general, people with Type II diabetes are at risk for all of the long-term complications seen with Type I. Therefore, it's important for you to be aware of the possible complications and to know what can be done to prevent them.

CHAPTER 12

DIABETES AND LARGE BLOOD VESSEL DISEASE

As you scan this chapter about the heart and blood vessel complications, you probably will recognize these problems as a concern for many Americans. And that is true. All Americans are at risk for large blood vessel disease, but people with diabetes have a greater reason to be concerned.

You need to know how diabetes affects your heart, how it affects your blood pressure, how it affects the blood vessels to your feet. We will define the problems and describe how to recognize them and how to treat them.

DIABETES AND YOUR HEART

Your heart could be called the most important organ in your body. It certainly could be considered the hardest working, beating on the average of 100,000 times a day.

A heart attack can be a major threat to the well-being of you and your heart. Certainly heart attacks are a concern for all people, whether they have diabetes or not, but we see two to four times the incidence of heart attack in people with diabetes compared with those without.

Heart attacks occur because of damage to the large blood vessels that supply the heart with nutrients and oxygen. If these blood vessels become blocked (as in coronary artery disease), damage can occur to the heart muscle. Injury to the blood vessels around the heart is caused by atherosclerosis—"hardening of the arteries." The process of atherosclerosis is not completely understood, but it is thought cholesterol plays a major role and diabetes and the related high blood glucose levels accelerate atherosclerosis.

Heart disease occurs at an earlier age in people with diabetes than in the general population. Women in the general population have a lower incidence of heart attacks until the time of menopause, while women with diabetes do not. In fact, the rate of heart attack is the same for men and women with diabetes, regardless of age.

Heart disease is characterized by a chest pain called angina. As the vessels that supply the heart become narrower, the heart muscle is damaged by a lack of oxygen and nutrients. This causes the pain. At first, the pain usually occurs when the person exercises or is active, when the heart has to work harder. However, as the heart muscle becomes more and more damaged, pain can occur at any time. Angina does not necessarily mean an individual is having a heart attack, but it is a warning of a serious problem. If nothing is done, a heart attack could occur.

Occasionally people with diabetes will have little or no chest pain and yet have a heart attack. These attacks are called "silent heart attacks". However, there may be other symptoms than chest pain that will tell you heart damage has taken place. These symptoms can include unexplained fatigue, shortness of breath, lesser tolerance for exercise and ankle swelling (edema). If you are having chest pain or other symptoms you think are related to your heart, see your doctor promptly.

HOW IS HEART DAMAGE ASSESSED?

There are a number of ways in which your heart health can be checked. The first test your doctor might order is an EKG (electrocardiogram). This is an electrical tracing of your heart's function at rest. Another test is a chest x-ray which can show your heart size and the possible presence of fluid in the lungs. If these tests are negative and there is still concern about the heart, a stress test may be done. This is an EKG done while you are exercising on a treadmill or exercise bike. If angina is severe and/or you have already had a heart attack, a cardiac catherization may be done. This is a study where dye is injected into the coronary arteries to see how much blockage is present. The results tell your doctor whether you may need treatment to replace or clear out the damaged arteries.

How can the blockage of arteries that supply the heart be reversed? There are a number of different ways to treat this problem. If you experience angina, see a doctor immediately for an evaluation and testing of the heart.

There are several medications available that could help expand the arteries to keep them open. Some people will need surgery—usually coronary artery bypass. With this procedure, blood vessels taken from the leg are used to bypass the blocked vessels near the heart.

Two newer techniques for treating coronary artery disease are available. One procedure is called "balloon angioplasty." After blockage has been established, a tube is inserted into the artery, a small balloon inflated and pulled back to expand the vessel. Another technique being pioneered is the use of a laser beam to open the blockage in the blood vessel.

DIABETES AND HIGH BLOOD PRESSURE

Almost two-thirds of adults with diabetes have high blood pressure—or hypertension.

As with some of the other problems discussed here, hypertension can occur in anyone, but it's more common in people with diabetes.

A number of factors can affect the incidence of hypertension in people with diabetes. Kidney damage is one; obesity is another. It's important to control blood pressure because the increased stress on blood vessels can speed the onset of other complications. And, of course, high blood pressure increases the risk for heart disease.

Because of the increased risk of heart, eye and kidney damage from high blood pressure, it is crucial that it be aggressively controlled in individuals with diabetes. Medication may be started sooner than in patients without diabetes. Treatment generally includes limiting your use of salt, controlling weight, and regular exercise in addition to medication.

A number of medications are available to treat high blood pressure. Many of these do have some side effects, and you may have to try a number of drugs before you find what works best for you. Because you have diabetes your doctor will need to carefully choose blood pressure medications that do not raise blood glucoses or fats or aggravate diabetes complications in other ways. Be aware of the importance of discussing all medications with your doctor whenever changes are made in your treatment plan.

DIABETES AND STROKE

Atherosclerosis in people with diabetes leads to a higher than normal incidence of stroke. Strokes are two to three times more common in people with diabetes than in the general population. Factors that can affect the incidence of stroke are high blood pressure and general health. Therefore, it's important to take control of your diabetes, monitor blood pressure, and maintain good health.

DIABETES AND POOR CIRCULATION TO THE LEGS

It is very common to see poor blood circulation to the legs (called Peripheral Vascular Disease or P.V.D.) in people with diabetes. This problem involves both the small and large blood vessels of the legs and feet. When the vessels become clogged, a person experiences discomfort or pain in the thigh or calf muscles while standing, walking or exercising. The first physical sign of loss of circulation may be the loss of pulses in the feet.

A good blood flow to the legs is always important but it becomes even more so when extra blood is needed to heal an injury or fight any infection that might occur in the foot.

Treatment of poor circulation can include the use of medication to improve blood flow. It is also possible to replace the damaged blood vessel with an artificial blood vessel.

HOW CAN ATHEROSCLEROSIS BE SLOWED OR PREVENTED?

A number of factors speed up the process of atherosclerosis. If these can be avoided or treated, the likelihood of serious problems with large and small blood vessels can be reduced. You can do a good deal to help prevent a heart attack or stroke.

The risk factors you can control include:

- Smoking
- High levels of cholesterol and triglycerides in the blood
- Obesity
- High blood pressure
- Blood glucose levels

(Diabetes itself is considered a risk factor
for heart disease and atherosclerosis.)

Smoking is a serious risk factor for both heart disease and blood vessel disease. People who smoke have two to four times the rate of vascular, or blood vessel disease as those who don't smoke. Therefore, if you now smoke, it is crucial to do everything possible to quit. If you have tried to quit without success, ask your doctor for referral to a reputable program that might help you succeed.

High blood levels of cholesterol have been associated with increased incidence of atherosclerosis and heart attack.

Studies have shown that a cholesterol level below 200 is optimal. It's interesting to note the low rate of heart disease in Japan where dietary fat intake is low compared with the high rate of heart disease in the United States and Finland—where fat intake is high. There are some people with family histories of high levels of triglycerides and cholesterol. Many of these people are at great risk for heart disease at a relatively early age. They not only need to follow a healthy, low-fat diet, but they also may need special medications.

Obesity is another risk factor for heart disease. In addition, people who are overweight may also have increased incidence of hypertension and poor control of diabetes. Therefore it's important to achieve and maintain a reasonable weight. (The level of obesity that is considered dangerous is 20 percent above one's ideal weight.)

High blood pressure have been mentioned several times, but it is so important to control blood pressure that it's worth mentioning again.

As we mentioned, diabetes is a risk factor for heart disease. The question is, does good blood glucose control play a role in preventing heart disease, as is the case with other complications? This has not been well researched, but some studies indicate improved blood glucose control may indeed slow the development of atherosclerosis.

WHAT YOU CAN DO

1. Do not smoke.
2. Strive for good control of diabetes.
3. See your doctor regularly for diabetes care.
4. Maintain a healthy weight.
5. Enjoy exercise as a regular part of your lifestyle.
6. Choose foods low in saturated fats and limit high cholesterol foods.
7. Choose foods low in sodium (salt).

WHAT YOUR DOCTOR CAN DO

1. Refer you to a "no smoking" program.
2. Check your blood pressure at each visit and begin an aggressive treatment plan if your blood pressure is elevated.
3. Test your blood annually for cholesterol and triglycerides.
4. Refer you to a registered dietitian or diabetes nutrition specialist for dietary guidance to lower cholesterol, fat and sodium in your diet, or lose weight if needed.
5. Order a hemoglobin A_1c and review this result and your blood glucose record to evaluate your control and adjust the treatment plan accordingly.
6. Test your heart function and circulation to all parts of your body with special emphasis on your feet at least annually if you are over 30 years old.

CHAPTER 13

DIABETES AND NERVE DAMAGE

One of the most marvelous systems of our body is the nervous system. Nerves are the communication system of the body—much like a network of telephone lines.

Nerves allow the brain to send messages to other parts of the body and the rest of the body to send messages back to the brain. Some nerves carry messages of sensation, such as pain, touch, or temperature. Others carry instructions from the brain to the legs, feet, hands, and internal organs. The nervous system is extensive, and its branches reach to every part of the body.

Damage to the nerves of the body is called neuropathy. When damage occurs to the nervous system, messages may become distorted or may not be communicated at all. The main cause of neuropathy appears to be high blood glucose levels damaging the nerves directly or being converted in the nerve to by-products which damage the nerve.

WHAT ARE THE SYMPTOMS?

Neuropathy does not always cause obvious symptoms, but when it does an individual may experience a loss of sensitivity or function in the affected area. Symptoms of neuropathy may develop gradually and then become suddenly worse. They may be severe for a while and then disappear.

Some symptoms of neuropathy may last for a few weeks to months, but in some cases the neuropathy may persist for months to years. On very rare occasions, symptoms may appear seemingly overnight and then disappear just as quickly.

WHAT NERVES ARE AFFECTED?

Perhaps the most common nerves affected in the body are those of the feet and lower legs. This neuropathy is characterized by numbness or tingling of the feet.

Eventually, a person could lose sensation in the feet, and no messages will be sent at all. A person could step on a sharp object and not even feel it.

Neuropathy also can affect nerves to organs and other body systems as well. Nerves to the penis are commonly affected, causing impotence in men. (See page 115.)

Another area where neuropathy can strike is nerves to the stomach and intestine, which in some people can cause severe constipation. In others, it can have the opposite effect, resulting in serious diarrhea. Neuropathy also can decrease one's ability to completely empty the bladder, which can lead to problems with bladder infections.

DETECTING NEUROPATHY

Your physician should check the function of your nerves as part of your routine diabetes care. This can be done by testing reflexes and checking your feet and hands for decreased sensation. Your physician should ask if you have trouble emptying your bladder, problems with impotence, or numbness, tingling, or unusual pain anywhere in your body. You can help prevent neuropathy by maintaining good blood glucose control.

If you have any problems with loss of feeling in any part of your body, such as your feet, it is important for you to take extra care to avoid injury to that area and to check daily for infections and other problems. And of course, be sure to tell your doctor about any problems you think may be developing.

HOW CAN NEUROPATHY BE TREATED?

Since high blood glucose levels are the main cause of neuropathy, the first line of treatment is to bring the blood glucoses as close to normal as possible. This often results in dramatic relief of painful neuropathy. Obtaining good glucose control is less likely to reverse the numbness some people experience but may help to slow the spread of this sensation (lack of feeling).

If achieving good control does not relieve the neuropathy, there are a number of other treatments to discuss with your health care team. Sometimes an anti depressant called amitriptyline (Elavil®) will be tried alone or in combination with another drug called fluphenazine (Prolixin®) to block the painful sensation of neuropathy.

In some individuals the pain is so severe that the use of pain medications may be needed for a short period of time. For most people, painful neuropathy is of short duration and will go away.

WHAT YOU CAN DO

1. Maintain good blood glucose control.
2. Tell your doctor about any tingling, numbness, loss of feeling, muscle weakness, pain or other unusual sensations.
3. Ask your doctor to investigate any persistent digestive or urinary problems.
4. If medications are prescribed, take them exactly as directed.

WHAT YOUR DOCTOR CAN DO

1. Order a hemoglobin A_1c test and review your blood glucose testing record to evaluate your blood glucose control and adjust the treatment plan accordingly.
2. Ask you regularly about symptoms of neuropathy.
3. Check the function of your nerves as part of routine diabetes care.
4. Refer you for diagnostic tests if symptoms occur.
5. Prescribe medication and pursue other methods of coping with painful neuropathy.
6. Teach you how to avoid problems which occur with loss of sensitivity, muscle weakness, and other possible effects of neuropathy.

CHAPTER 14

CARING FOR YOUR FEET

Most ordinary people think having sore feet is a normal part of life. They accept the discomfort and don't pay much attention to it. They go on putting their feet into tight, narrow, pointed, thin-soled shoes and wearing tight, slippery synthetic stockings, thinking that painful feet are the price that must be paid to be stylish. They ignore their feet and usually suffer only minor problems as a result.

People with diabetes, though, aren't ordinary—they're special. If you have diabetes, high-fashion shoes and stockings are not just painful, they are bad for your feet. It's currently estimated that there are 30,000-40,000 amputations each year among Americans who have diabetes. Experts think half to three-quarters of these amputations can be avoided with proper foot care.

SPECIAL CARE IS NEEDED

There are three reasons why people with diabetes are at high risk for foot problems.

• The first is decreased circulation to the legs and feet. (See Chapter 12.)

• A second reason is the loss of the sensation in the feet. (See Chapter 13.)

• The third reason for concern is a decreased ability to fight infection when diabetes is poorly controlled.

These three problems often work together to make even a common occurance like a callous, a threat to your health. Because of loss of feeling, you may not be aware of a callous forming. As it becomes thicker, the tissue under the callous can be damaged. If the skin is very dry, cracking can occur, allowing bacteria to enter. Infection can easily develop. When there is decreased circulation or poor control of blood glucose, it will be very hard for the body to fight this infection.

Without prompt treatment there is serious risk of further damaging the tissue to create a condition called gangrene. If this happens it is not reversible and the only treatment is amputation.

In most cases, however, serious foot problems can be prevented. Keeping your blood glucoses well controlled is crucial for general foot health and healing. You must also make foot care a part of your daily routine. Follow these guidelines:

DO

1. Inspect your feet daily for cracks, blisters, infections, and injuries. You may be able to see a problem before you feel it. If you can't see the bottoms of your feet easily, use a mirror. A magnifying glass also may help you see better. If you can't check your own feet, have someone do it for you.

2. Cleanse your feet daily as you bathe or shower, using warm water and mild soap. Dry your feet with a soft towel, making sure to dry between the toes.

3. Moisturize dry skin by using an emollient cream that contains urea. If it causes redness or irritation, discontinue it's use and inform your doctor. If you are currently using a cream or lotion that keeps your skin soft and free of cracks, continue using it.

4. Clip toenails straight across. If you are bothered by sharp toenail edges, use a cardboard emory board to smooth down the edges. If you can't easily reach your feet or have thick nails, have a podiatrist trim your nails.

5. Always wear something on your feet to protect from injury—even in your house.

6. Choose good shoes. Wear socks that are a cotton or wool blend. We recommend that women wear a cotton "footlet" inside nylons or purchase cotton-soled nylons.

CHARACTERISTICS OF A GOOD SHOE

- Soft leather upper
- Soft insole and inner lining, free of rough areas and thick seams
- Firm sole
- Length: 1/2 inch longer than your longest toe when standing
- Toe box: wide and shaped like your foot

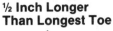

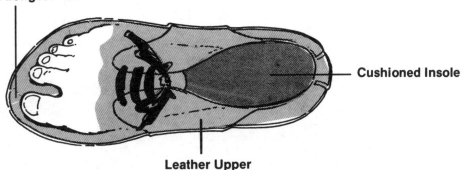

½ Inch Longer Than Longest Toe

Cushioned Insole

Leather Upper

7. Treat minor breaks in the skin promptly. Cleanse the area with soap and water, dry, and cover with clean gauze. Observe for signs of infection such as redness, swelling, warmth, pain, or drainage. Stay off of the foot until you have further evaluation or instruction from your doctor.

8. See your doctor promptly for foot injuries. Stay off your foot until it is evaluated by the doctor.

9. Ask your doctor to check your feet during your regular visits for diabetes care. Take off your shoes and socks at every visit. At some point you may require referral to a foot care specialist or podiatrist for help with ingrown toenails, corns, callouses, trimming thick toenails, or if you need specially fitted shoes.

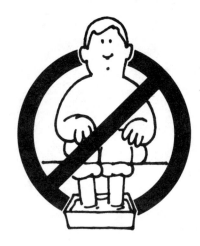

DON'T

1. **DO NOT** soak your feet.
—Soaking dries skin excessively, creating cracks. This allows bacteria to enter, possibly causing infections. Also, soaking will delay the healing process.

2. **DO NOT** use hot water bottles or heating pads or any electrical device for heating or stimulating the feet.

3. **DO NOT** use a pumice stone to remove callouses. This will stimulate further callous formation.

4. **DO NOT** smoke. Smoking reduces blood flow to the feet in addition to causing many other health hazards.

5. **DO NOT** wear tight fitting shoes or stockings. They restrict blood flow to the feet. For the same reason, avoid sitting with your legs crossed.

6. **DO NOT** use commercial wart or corn removers on your feet.

7. **DO NOT** perform "bathroom surgery" by using razor blades or other sharp instruments on your feet.

8. **DO NOT** minimize a foot problem, however minor it may seem.

WHAT YOUR DOCTOR CAN DO

1. Check your feet at each regular diabetes care visit.
2. Ask if you are having any foot problems or leg pains.
3. Check the pulses in your legs and feet.
4. Check your ability to feel light touch, vibrations, and pain in your feet and legs.
5. Check for callouses, cuts, bruises, infections, bunions, ulcers, and ingrown toenails.
6. All doctors are not created equally interested in diabetes foot care, so be sure you find a doctor who is concerned about proper foot care. You need and deserve the best care you can get!

CHAPTER 15

IMPOTENCE: A COMMON PROBLEM

Impotence is defined as the inability to achieve or maintain an erection suitable to complete a successful act of sexual intercourse. It's true that any man may have trouble with impotence at one time or another but it occurs much more frequently in men with diabetes. In fact studies indicate that up to 50 percent of men with diabetes will eventually have problems with sexual function.

To understand how diabetes causes impotence, it's helpful to understand how the body produces an erection. A normal erection requires a fairly complicated series of events. First the man must be sexually excited. Then a series of signals passes from the brain along the nerves to the blood vessels in the penis. This causes spongy tissue within the penis to fill with blood and expand. This expansion then produces a shaft that is stiff enough to allow insertion into the vagina. The erection must be maintained until orgasm and ejaculation occur. Problems at any stage of this process can cause impotence.

The main problem in diabetes is damage to the nerves that carry the signals to the blood vessels of the penis. If these nerve signals are blocked the penis does not expand and there is no erection. Impotence related to diabetes is usually not reversible. It generally develops slowly over many months to years. Erections become softer and less frequent until there's total inability to achieve or maintain an erection.

If you experience impotence, you should see your doctor for a complete medical evaluation of the problem. Just because you have diabetes does not mean that's the cause of your impotence. There are other causes of impotence—both psychological and physical.

WHAT IS THE TREATMENT?

New methods of treatment have been developed to make erection and intercourse possible again.

Two main types of treatment are available. One involves injection of drugs into the penis. These drugs increase the blood flow into the penis and the result is an erection that lasts from 20-60 minutes. This method of obtaining an erection does not work for all men with diabetes, but it has been helpful for many.

A second approach to treatment is surgery involving a penile prosthesis. This is a device implanted into the penis to provide sufficient rigidity for intercourse. The device does not interfere with urination or ejaculation. There are three types of prostheses now available: the semi-rigid, the maleable, and the inflatable. The choice of which prosthesis is most appropriate for the individual depends on many factors that should be discussed with your physician and a urologist who is expert in this type of surgery. Studies of men who have been treated with implants have revealed that more than 90 percent are satisfied with the device.

For any treatment of impotence to be successful, the man and his partner should both be involved in deciding the most appropriate treatment.

CHAPTER 16

KEEPING AN EYE ON YOUR EYES

What a marvelous creation our eyes are. We take them for granted and often choose not to think about what it would be like to lose our vision. And yet we have heard the frightening statistics about diabetes and eye disease or blindness. Overwhelming as this information might be, it only reflects the past. Today, it need not be as threatening as it once was.

New diagnostic tests and treatment can help us maintain healthy eyes to a much greater extent than was possible even a few years ago. Regular yearly—or sometimes more frequent—eye exams can help detect eye problems before they progress too far. This means your doctor can treat the problem before you lose precious sight.

RETINOPATHY

The retina is the area of the eye where light changes into electrical impulses that are sent to the brain. Damage to this area is called retinopathy. About half of all people who have had diabetes more than 10 years develop diabetic retinopathy. The figure climbs to 80 percent in those who have had diabetes more than 25 years.

For reasons we don't fully understand, diabetes can damage blood vessels throughout our bodies. The vessels in the eyes seem especially vulnerable to damage. In the early stages of retinopathy, called background retinopathy, the small blood vessels in the retina can leak fluid. If this leaking occurs in the macula, then objects may appear blurry. (The macula is the center of the retina which controls our sharp reading vision.)

Proliferative retinopathy is an advanced form of retinopathy. About 10 percent of people with diabetes have this condition. It's even more common in those who have had diabetes from 15 to 20 years or longer. Proliferative retinopathy occurs when abnormal blood vessels grow on the retina and sometimes into other parts of the eye. If these vessels bleed into the vitreous, the clear fluid in the center of the eye, light can't reach the retina and vision can become cloudy. The blood may be slowly reabsorbed and vision can return to normal. But if the bleeding continues, vision may be cloudy until the problem is treated.

Tissue can also grow along with the abnormal blood vessels, distorting vision or making objects appear blurry. Over time, the tissue can shrink, pulling the retina away from its base.

If the blood doesn't reabsorb or if the tissue affects your vision, the vitreous may need to be surgically removed to avoid loss of vision.

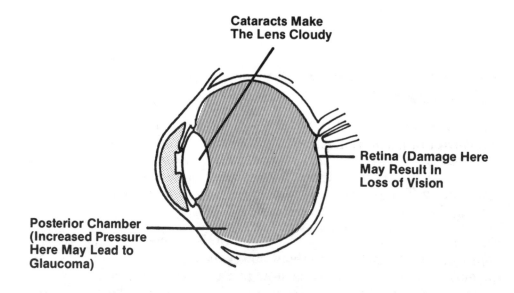

DETECTING THE PROBLEM

When you go the the doctor for an eye exam, he or she will check your retina using one of several methods.

Your pupils will be dilated and the eye specialist will check the retina with a device called an ophthalmoscope, which directs a beam of light into your eye to look at the blood vessels in the back of the eye.

A slit lamp, a microscope used to magnify the inside of the eye, is another tool your doctor might use to examine your eyes. Again, your eyes are dilated and a lens is held near your eye so the doctor can see the eye in detail.

If the retina looks suspicious, your doctor might want to do a fluorescein angiogram. A dye called fluorescein is injected into your arm, taking only a few seconds to reach the eyes. As the dye travels through the blood vessels in the eyes, technicians take several photographs of your retina. These photographs will show if any leakage or abnormal blood vessels are present. Your doctor will know exactly what areas of the retina need to be treated.

WHAT CAN BE DONE?

If your fluorescein angiogram shows leakage affecting or threatening vision, your doctor will probably prescribe laser treatment. The laser is a very small, intense light beam. The doctor aims the laser at the leaking vessels and seals the leaks. But laser treatment may not stop leakage in new areas. Therefore, it isn't a permanent cure for retinopathy.

The effect of laser treatment on your vision can vary. Sometimes it helps restore lost vision, while other times it may only keep vision from getting worse. In some people it slows down the progression of eye disease. A lot depends on how early eye changes are detected and treated. Proliferative retinopathy is best treated in the early stages.

Be sure your blood pressure is well controlled. Any elevation in blood pressure can increase the leaking in already damaged small blood vessels.

That's why it's so important for you to have your eyes checked at least once a year. If you do have vision problems, your doctor will probably want to see you more often— maybe every three to four months.

As with most aspects of diabetes management, you're the key player on your health care team. Please pay attention to your vision. If you notice any changes, call your doctor right away.

WHAT YOU CAN DO

1. Carefully control the amount of glucose in your blood—if it remains high keep in close contact with your doctor.
2. See your doctor for diabetes care regularly (2-4 times a year).
3. Have your eyes dilated and examined closely at least once a year.
4. See an ophthalmologist promptly if eye changes are found.

Remember, YOU are the most important person caring for your diabetes. Your actions and those of your doctor may save your vision.

WHAT YOUR DOCTOR CAN DO:

1. Ask you if you have any vision problems at each visit.
2. Put drops in your eyes to dilate and examine them at least once a year.
3. Have you read an eye chart at least once each year.
4. Have you see an eye specialist (ophthalmologist) at least once a year.
5. Check your blood presure at each visit and if it is consistently high, start treatment right away.
6. If changes are found in your eyes, have you see an eye specialist who can treat them with laser or other methods.

CHAPTER 17

THE KIDNEYS—NATURE'S MARVELOUS FILTER

The kidneys are a pair of organs whose job is to filter the blood to remove waste products of the body's functions. The kidneys are made up of millions of closely packed small blood vessels that carry the blood through the kidneys, where it is filtered. In people with poorly controlled diabetes, the kidneys must constantly filter large amounts of glucose out of the blood.

People who develop diabetes early in life (before age 20) have a high risk of kidney damage, and in the past about half of these people had kidney disease after 15 to 20 years. People with Type II diabetes have a lower risk of kidney disease. It is thought that this rate can be lowered greatly by good control of diabetes.

CONTROL MAKES A DIFFERENCE

The first thing you must do to help protect your kidneys is to keep your blood glucose levels as close to normal as possible. This will allow the small kidney blood vessels to filter the blood without being damaged. If your blood glucose levels are high most of the time, you will increase your chances of suffering serious kidney disease.

SYMPTOMS AND SIGNS OF KIDNEY DISEASE

Usually the first indication of damage to the kidney, due to diabetes, is the appearance of protein (mostly albumin) in the urine. The protein, which we all carry in our blood, leaks through the damaged glomeruli, or small filtering tubes, and appears in the urine. It is detected when your doctor does a routine urine protein test. The presence of protein in the urine produces no discomfort and the person is not aware of its presence unless the urine is tested.

As the amount of protein lost into the urine increases, the level of it in the blood falls below the normal range. Then some of the water in the blood vessels seeps into the tissue under the skin to produce a swelling called edema.

As damage to the small blood vessels continues to progress, the kidneys will have more and more problems getting rid of waste products.

Another test that measures the level of waste products in the blood is called a creatinine test. If damage continues— the kidneys will stop working. Then the alternatives are renal dialysis or a kidney transplant.

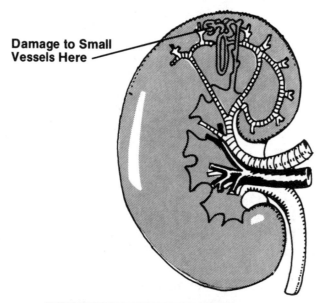

Damage to Small Vessels Here

WATCH BLOOD PRESSURE

An important way you can help your kidneys is to take steps to prevent high blood pressure (hypertension) and to treat it right away if it develops. High blood pressure causes damage to small blood vessels. When you have diabetes, high blood pressure adds to the damage that high blood glucose can cause in the small blood vessels of the kidney.

Make certain your blood pressure is checked each time you see your doctor. If he or she finds you consistently have blood pressures of 140/90 or higher, a prescription drug is indicated in addition to the recommendations in Chapter 12.

Some studies would indicate that drug treatment should be started at a lower level (135/85).

BEWARE OF INFECTION

Another way you can protect your kidneys is to be on the alert for kidney and bladder infections.

A bladder infection usually produces an urge to urinate frequently. This may be every 15 to 30 minutes—sometimes more often. Urination may be painful, and sometimes the urine is bloody. An infection of one or both kidneys produces back pain near the lowest ribs, chills, high fever, and often cloudy urine.

If you have any of these signs, see your doctor right away. A urine sample will be checked. If you have an infection, your doctor may prescribe a drug to treat it.

WHAT YOU CAN DO

1. Work with your doctor to control your diabetes and keep blood glucose levels as close to normal as possible.
2. Guard against high blood pressure by cutting back on the amount of sodium (salt) you eat, losing weight if necessary, and exercising regularly.
3. Have high blood pressure treated right away if it develops.
4. Be on the lookout for kidney and bladder infections and have them treated right away.

WHAT YOUR DOCTOR
CAN DO

1. Check your diabetes control by reviewing your record book and doing the hemoglobin A_1c test and adjusting the treatment if needed.
2. Check your blood pressure at each visit and recommend ways you can prevent or treat high blood pressure.
3. Check a urine sample at least once a year for protein. If signs of possible damage are found, doing further tests as indicated.
4. Ask you about symptoms of kidney and urinary infections.
5. Refer you to a specialist if kidney damage develops.

CHAPTER 18

MOTIVATION—KEEPING YOURSELF MOVING

Motivation is the "force" in our lives that leads to action. The word itself stems from motive—something that causes a person to act. It's motivation that moves us from knowing what needs to be done to doing it. We can gather lots of information about diabetes, for example, but unless we are motivated to do something with that information nothing changes. Motivation is the key ingredient that leads to action.

What can we do to improve our motivation? One "tool" is positive coping. Robert Lewis Stevenson, who had tuberculosis, once said, "Life is not a matter of getting a good hand, but of playing a poor hand well." We can't always control what happens in our lives, but we certainly can control how we cope with it.

SKILLS FOR COPING

Positive coping involves a number of skills—skills people can learn and then apply. The first skill is information gathering. That's what you are doing by reading this book, attending a class or asking questions.

A second step is setting realistic goals. We often set goals that are too high. We may even expect ourselves to be perfect. As a result, we set ourselves up to fail.

Think about your own experience. How often have you expected yourself to stick to a diet that was too rigid and too restrictive? You expected too much of yourself. Setting goals that are realistic for you allows you to experience success rather than failure.

A third skill is problem solving. Often we think about all the things we have to do, and we become overwhelmed. Problem solving has to do with breaking down goals, taking a look at the obstacles that stand in our way to accomplishing these goals and overcoming those obstacles.

Yet another aspect of coping is taking direct action, being assertive, taking risks, and communicating our needs. This can be difficult. Sometimes it's hard to ask for the kind of support you want from your family and friends.

Another skill in coping is managing stress effectively. Thinking about diabetes can be stressful, and the expectations we place on ourselves also add stress to our lives. We might consider lowering the expectations we have of ourselves by setting more realistic goals. We can also read about stress management and learn to relax. One of the easiest ways to relax is to take a long walk.

One final form of positive coping is the use of humor. Mary Pettibone Poole said, "He who laughs, lasts!" Laughter is like internal jogging. It's not simply telling a good story or joke; rather it's an approach to life.

YOU CAN MAKE CHOICES

In addition to positive coping, we can be motivated by choice. Think about the serenity prayer: *"God grant me the courage to accept the things I cannot change, the strength to change the things I can, and the wisdom to distinguish between the two."*

There are a lot of things in life we can't change. You didn't ask for diabetes, but you have it. However, there are so many choices available to you to help you deal with your diabetes. It's your choice whether or not to test your blood glucose or to make changes in your eating and exercise habits. That choice will determine how well you live with diabetes.

Take Jean for instance. She thought of all the things she felt she *should* do. She *should* exercise daily, she *should* stick to her diet, she *should* finish all those projects she had piled up at home—the list went on and on. Sometimes we choose to do too much. A good saying to help you avoid doing that is, *"Thou shalt not **should** on thyself."*

It helps to make a list of all the things you think you "should" do. From that list, pick one or two that you "choose" to work on. When you change *should* to *choose* you change procrastination and excuses into action. In Jean's case, she chose to walk five minutes every day—a realistic goal and one she could succeed at. She also chose to change from whole milk to 1% milk.

Remember, you can't change everything at once. Just feeling you are making specific choices can give you renewed motivation to put those choices into action.

SEEK SUPPORT

Accepting your feelings is the step that follows identifying and communicating those feelings. If you feel support from those around you, it will help you accept those feelings.

Just as there are many different feelings, there are many different ways to deal with those feelings. We all need different kinds of support as we learn to live with diabetes. You may be connected with many different support systems—family, church, work, clubs—and perhaps you don't particularly need any new or different groups to feel supported in dealing with diabetes. On the other hand, you may experience a dramatic need for support related specifically to diabetes because there are very few people without diabetes who understand what it's like. It's important you seek out what's right for you.

Another reason to find support is to maintain motivation. We all know how hard it is to be motivated for everyday tasks. Controlling diabetes requires a lot of motivation because you are the only one responsible for it. It's easy to become discouraged, to forget or to give up. It may help to keep in mind that diabetes is a disease of self-management and your support needs are part of that self-management.

BELIEFS

Closely related to feelings are our beliefs. These are simply our own concepts of what something means—what we believe about ourselves or about the world. Beliefs affect how we behave, and what we believe about diabetes affects how we will do in controlling it. If we believe, for example, that we are incapable of making changes in our lives, then we are likely not to make any changes.

Mark had this problem when he was told to lose weight. Since he had never been successful at losing weight before, he believed he was unable to succeed. With this belief in mind, he was setting himself up not to make any changes.

Mark's thought process went something like this: "I am unable to lose weight, which means my diabetes will not be under control, which means I am not going to live a healthy life with diabetes, which leaves me feeling helpless, hopeless, powerless and ashamed. I am the one who is responsible—yet there is no way I can change."

If Mark had continued to think this way, he would probably have made no changes and would have felt awful about his failure. In the end, he probably would not have lived a very healthy life with diabetes.

We all have beliefs about what keeps us well, what makes us ill and what we need to do to get better. Dr. Marshall Becker at the University of Michigan says individuals will only stick to a medical plan if they (1) believe their condition is serious or severe; (2) believe the condition or complications of that condition can happen to them; and (3) believe the benefit of sticking to a treatment plan will outweigh the costs.

As you learn diabetes is serious, you probably will become more motivated to take care of yourself and to stick to your management plan. As you learn about the benefits of taking good care of yourself, you may decide the benefits of blood testing, staying with your diet and exercising outweigh the costs—the financial costs, the extra time you have to spend taking care of yourself and the things you might give up.

BEWARE OF KILLER PHRASES

Beliefs about ourselves also dramatically affect our behavior. We all give ourselves messages all the time. Too often, these messages are negative: "You're too lazy." "You're too fat." "You should have done a better job." "You can't do that."

These messages are called "killer phrases" because they erode our self-esteem and make us less effective, less happy, and less able to take care of ourselves.

Negative messages often become a habit. We need to practice giving ourselves positive affirmations that we are capable, that we deserve happiness, praise, love, and that we can learn about diabetes, take control of the situation and live well. Practice these affirmations. You might feel silly at first, but they will have a positive effect.

A final set of beliefs that affect how we live well with diabetes is our belief about the world and most specifically about *hope*. For people without hope, behavior change and positive self-management are pointless. It is only with a sense of hope that people can move on to do the things they need to do for themselves.

CHAPTER 19

ACTION!

Now that we've given you page after page of information, you have the option of doing something with it—of putting together your personal plan for action.

This plan begins with a goal. In the broadest sense, that goal is to live well. You need to decide what that means in your life. Zero in on some very specific ways to move toward a healthier lifestyle.

By carefully looking at what you are doing now—your behaviors—you can plan for change. And that change need not, in fact probably should not, be dramatic. Small steps may take longer, but you won't tend to be so overwhelmed along the way that you lose your enthusiasm.

If you're using this book as part of a class experience, there might be someone sitting next to you right now who will say, "What's the big deal. I'll lose 50 pounds in two months, start running three miles a day, eat three balanced, calorie controlled meals and two snacks every day, check my blood glucose religiously, three times a day every day, take a stress management course, join a health club . . . " You might feel intimidated by such self discipline, but don't be misled. Those goals are far too ambitious for 99 percent of the mortals of this world. Superperson, yes. Joe Smith, no.

Make your personal goals reachable!! Set yourself up to succeed. Choose to lose a pound a week and walk six blocks a day, four days a week. Then do it—and reward yourself for a good job.

We'll all encounter obstacles. We're tired after a hard day at work and don't feel like exercising. We don't want to bother with meal plans. The idea of sticking your finger is just too much some days. Write down those obstacles that most likely will get in the way of your success.

Support is also important. You're going to need lots of encouragement as you make changes. Write down your sources of support. Friends, family, social groups. Do you have an internal support also—a faith that helps you gain inner strength? List all of them and plan how you might use them to reach your goal of living well.

Think about the signs that warn you you're off track. What behaviors creep in when you're slipping off the track? Do you start to skip exercise? Do you avoid your health care team? Do you forget to take your medication? Write these things down also and be sensitive to when they occur in your day-to-day life. When you find yourself doing these things, have a chat with yourself.

We hope you will design your own, very specific action plan. To get you started here are some guidelines.

- Choose action items from these general areas. Identify what your specific concern is.

  > Exercise
  > Meal planning
  > Losing weight
  > Taking medication regularly
  > Monitoring blood glucose levels
  > Emotional health
  > Other _____

- Identify what you can do differently. Answer these questions.

  > What?
  > When?
  > Where?
  > How often?
  > With whom?

- Know for sure that you can meet these goals, then DO it!

MY SELF ASSESSMENT

Action begins by identifying a problem behavior. What is the problem? Is it one of doing something too much or not enough?

_____

_____

_____

What situations or places trigger the problem behavior?

_____

_____

What are the payoffs for not changing?

_____

_____

What are the payoffs for changing?

_____

_____

Who supports this behavior change?

_____

_____

Who hinders this behavior change?

_____

_____

Are you ready to change? If so, move on to fill out your action plan.

MY ACTION PLAN

MY GOAL:

Two week objective: (What can I realistically do in the next 2 weeks?)

What: _____
_____
_____

When: _____
_____
_____

Where: _____
_____
_____

How often: _____
_____
_____

With whom: _____
_____
_____

Two weeks later: Did I meet my objective?

☐ YES: My next 2 week objective:

_____
_____
_____

☐ NO: What were my obstacles?

_____
_____

What am I willing to do differently to overcome these obstacles in the next 2 weeks?

_____
_____
_____

As you can see, this is an continuous process: looking at where you want to go, taking steps to get there, checking on our progress and resetting goals.

An important aspect of living well is flexibility. Be prepared for weak moments—and forgive yourself quickly when you have a slip. Also, don't forget to live life with a sense of humor. If a healthier lifestyle becomes a burden, you're not likely to be excited about it. Choose what you enjoy and then enjoy what you choose.

CHAPTER 20

A LOOK AT THE FUTURE: DIABETES RESEARCH

What lies ahead in terms of new treatments for people with diabetes? Is there a cure on the horizon?

You may have heard about the possibility of pancreas transplants or the transplantation of insulin-producing beta cells that will provide a source of insulin for people with diabetes. Research is continuing on these approaches, and great advances have been seen. However, these treatments are primarily for individuals with Type I diabetes in whom the pancreas is not producing insulin.

For most people with Type II diabetes, insulin is available, but it doesn't work as it should. While pancreas transplants could possibly be helpful in supplying extra insulin, this insulin may not work well either. As we look at ways to cure Type II diabetes, we need to concentrate on what can be done to make insulin work as it should.

DRUG RESEARCH IS MOVING AHEAD

One approach involves investigating different types of drugs that help insulin work better. There are a number of agents being tried experimentally, and scientists are hopeful some of these will enhance insulin's action.

Another area in which research continues involves new ways to help people lose weight and maintain that weight loss. We know when people are obese, they need more insulin and that insulin often doesn't work well. Therefore, if a person with Type II diabetes can lose weight, insulin may be able to do its job once again.

KEEPING GLUCOSE LEVELS IN LINE

Research also is underway to find agents to return blood glucose levels to normal and prevent damage to blood vessels. Along these lines, investigators are studying how to block the effect of glucose, which may lead to ways to prevent some of the complications associated with diabetes.

Among the agents being tested are the aldose reductase inhibitors, which block the conversion of glucose into a sugar called sorbitol. This sugar has been linked with damage to blood vessels in some instances.

PREVENTION IS THE FIRST PRIORITY

At this point, prevention of complications is a major goal. Control of blood glucose levels appears to be a major key, and a national study is currently documenting the value of control, particulary in Type I diabetes.

In the meantime, new methods of treating diabetes complications are also being tested. One study is looking at the best time to start laser treatment to help reduce eye damage. New methods of testing and evaluating the heart are being sought. Even if there may not be a definitive cure for Type II diabetes on the horizon, the future looks promising.

EDUCATION IS THE KEY INGREDIENT

One final reminder. Unless individuals learn how to take care of their diabetes and how to find reliable sources of information and appropriate health care, efforts at prevention and treatment will be of little value. It's important that this message reach people with Type II diabetes. You need to know as much as you possibly can about the disease and its care. And remember, information is constantly changing. Check with your health care team often to learn what's new.

HERE'S TO YOUR HEALTHIER LIFE

This *Invitation to a Healthier Lifestyle* has been prepared for you by a group of folks who have seen what people can do to turn their lives around. We hope we have given you some new tools for healthy living, some motivation for success, and some zest for the years ahead.

INDEX

If you found this book helpful and would like more information on this and other related subjects you may be interested in one or more of the following titles from our *Wellness and Nutrition Library.*

BOOKS

NUTRITION

The Joy of Snacks: Good nutrition for people who like to snack (270 pages)
Pass the Pepper Please: For people on sodium restricted diets (70 pages)
Fast Food Facts: Nutritive and exchange values for fast food restaurants (56 pages)
Convenience Food Facts: Help for the healthy meal planner (216 pages)
Opening the Door to Good Nutrition (186 pages)
A Guide to Healthy Eating: Facts about fat, cholesterol, fiber and salt (60 pages)
The Guiltless Gourmet: Recipes, menus and nutritional information for the health conscious cook (147 pages)
Eating With Food Choices (44 pages)

WELLNESS

I Can Cope: Staying Healthy With Cancer (216 pages)
The Physician Within: Taking charge of your well being (175 pages)
Learning to Live Well with Diabetes (392 pages)
Exchanges for All Occasions: Meeting the challenge of diabetes (210 pages)
Managing the School Age Child with a Chronic Health Condition: A practical guide for schools, families and organizations (284 pages)
Managing Type II Diabetes: Your invitation to a healthier lifestyle (170 pages)

BOOKLETS & PAMPHLETS

Diabetes & Alcohol (4 pages)
Diabetes & Exercise (20 pages)
Emotional Adjustment to Diabetes (16 pages)
Healthy Footsteps for People with Diabetes (13 pages)
Diabetes Record Book (68 pages)
Diabetes & Brief Illness (8 pages)
Diabetes & Impotence: A concern for Couples (6 pages)
Adding Fiber to Your Diet (16 pages)
Gestational Diabetes: Guidelines for a Safe Pregnancy and Healthy Baby (36 pages)
Recognizing and Treating Insulin Reactions (4 pages)
Hypoglycemia (functional) (4 pages)

SPECIFICALLY FOR THE HEALTH PROFESSIONAL

Low Literacy Series: 17 booklets for teaching diabetes management with low literacy skills
Youth Curriculum: For working with young diabetic patients, ages 6 to 16

The *Wellness and Nutrition Library* is published by DCI Publishing, a division of Diabetes Center, Inc., in Minneapolis, Minnesota, publishers of quality educational materials dealing with health, wellness, nutrition, diabetes and other chronic illnesses. All our books and materials are available nationwide and in Canada through leading bookstores. If you are unable to find our books at your favorite bookstore, contact us directly for a free catalog.

DCI Publishing
P. O. Box 739
Wayzata, MN 55391